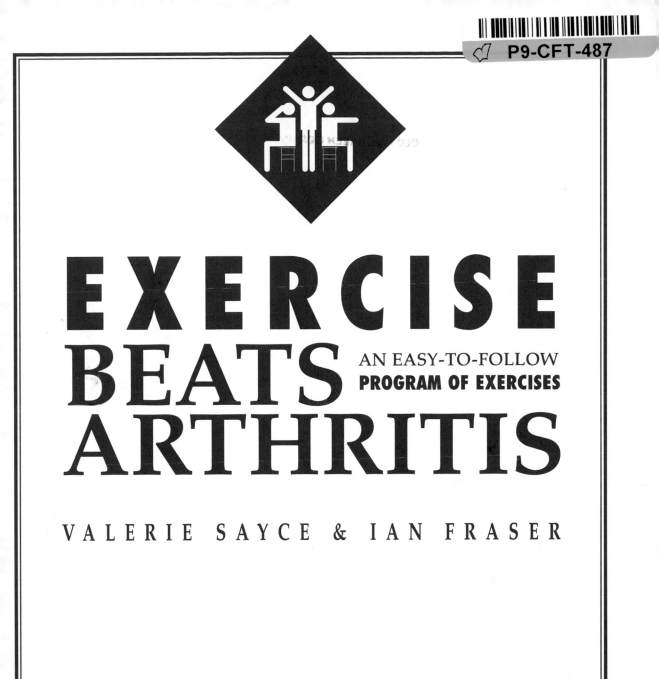

EXERCISE
BEATS
AN EASY-TO-FOLLOW
PROGRAM OF EXERCISES
ARTHRITIS

VALERIE SAYCE & IAN FRASER

BULL PUBLISHING

Copyright © 1998 Bull Publishing Company

Bull Publishing Company
P. O. Box 208
Palo Alto, CA 94302-0208
Phone (650) 322-2855
Fax (650) 327-3300
www.bullpub.com

ISBN 0-923521-45-3

Distributed in the United States by:
Publishers Group West
1700 Fourth Street
Berkeley, CA 94710

Publisher: James Bull
Production: Publication Services, Inc.
Cover Design: Robb Pawlak, Pawlak Design
Interior Design: Publication Services, Inc.
Printer: Malloy Lithographing, Inc.
All updated photographs for this edition by R. C. Adams

Sayce, Valerie.
    Exercise beats arthritis. / Valerie Sayce, Ian Fraser.—3rd ed.
        p.   cm.
    Includes bibliographical references and index.
    ISBN 0-923521-45-3
    1. Arthritis—Exercise therapy.   I. Fraser, Ian, 1936–   .
  II. Title.
  RC933.S26   1998
  616.7'22062–dc21   98-30859
                                                      CIP

10 9 8 7 6 5 4 3 2

Contents

1 **What Is Arthritis?** 1
Rheumatoid Arthritis 2
Osteoarthritis 4
Ankylosing Spondylitis 7
Neck and Low Back Pain 7
Bursitis and Tendonitis 8
Fibromyalgia Syndrome 9
Osteoporosis 10

2 **Let's Find Out About** 15
Diet 15
Mental Attitude 17
Stress 17
Visiting the Doctor 17
Medication 18
Other Health Professionals 19
Surgery 20
Comfort Techniques 20
Joint Protection 20
The Weather 21

3 **Your Exercise Program** 23
Why Exercise 23
Types of Exercise 24
Exercise with Care 24
Who Should Exercise 25
What to Exercise 25
When to Exercise 26
Where to Exercise 26
What to Wear 26
Before You Exercise 26
How to Exercise 27
After You Exercise 27
Planning Your Exercise Program 27
Maintaining Motivation 30
Points to Remember 32

4 **Morning Wake Up** 33

5 **Warm Up** 43

6 **Neck** 49

7 **Arms** 53

8 **Hands** 59

9 **Back** 65

10 **Hips** 79

11 **Knees** 85

12 **Feet** 91

13 **Cool Down** 97

14 **Water Exercise** 103

v

15 **Aerobic Exercise** 115
Getting Started   116
Determining Exercise Intensity   116
Building Up   117
Warm Up and Cool Down   117
Specific Aerobic Activities   117
Exercise Opportunities   118

16 **Relaxation** 119
Methods of Relaxation   120
Relaxation and Sleep   122

17 **Using Your Body** 125
Posture   126
Getting Up from a Chair   128
Lifting   129
Getting Down to and
   Up from the Floor   130
Everyday Efficiency   131

Further Reading 96

Index 133

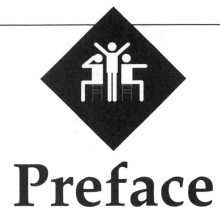

Preface

Learning to Live with It

Arthritis and rheumatism are general terms that cover a wide range of joint problems and other aches and pains. Most of us experience something of the kind at some time in our lives. It is only when the symptoms linger, or if they are particularly painful, that we seek advice and help from our doctor.

You may already have sought help. Perhaps you got good advice, or maybe you were told, "Oh, you've just got a bit of arthritis. Here is something for the pain. Not much we can do-you'll just have to learn to live with it."

This presents a rather hopeless picture, doesn't it? You think your pain and suffering have not been taken seriously. However, it is not true that nothing can be done. Think carefully about the words "learn to live with it." This is actually good advice.

"Learning to live with it" does not mean that you withdraw from life for fear of doing anything that might aggravate your condition. This will only lead to you feeling miserable and sorry for yourself. Nor does it mean the other extreme of deliberately ignoring what your body is saying to you in an attempt to maintain your normal lifestyle. Rather, you must find a balance whereby you learn to live with your arthritis. You learn to recognize, listen, and respond to your body's signals.

A good starting point is to find out about the type of arthritis you have and what it is doing to your body. Become more aware, also, of what your body is telling you: what makes you feel worse and what makes you feel better. And, above all, recognize that there is a lot you can do to help yourself. The more understanding you have of your problem, the better you will be able to manage your arthritis. You can still lead a satisfying and enjoyable life.

So how can *Exercise Beats Arthritis* help you achieve this aim? Arthritis is primarily a disease that affects your joints and their support structures. Exercises use those joints and muscles, so it's in your power to work directly on your problems.

Different exercises have different purposes. As you will find through reading this book and practicing the exercises, there are many ways in which exercises can have beneficial effects.

Exercise is one of the most useful and direct ways in which you can help minimize the pain and the limitations of arthritis. However, be careful with what type of exercise you do. It is possible to make your problems worse with injudicious exercises. By working through this book, you will be able to develop an appropriate and beneficial exercise program for you and your arthritis.

Acknowledgments

Our thanks are due to the many people who helped or contributed to this book in different ways. Dr. Danny Lewis, a rheumatologist who has long been involved with the Arthritis Foundation of Victoria (AFV) evaluated the exercise sequences and provided several helpful suggestions that, in the end, made the book better. Jenny Davidson, the AFV's former programs manager, drew generously from her expertise on many occasions during the books' embryonic and developmental phases, and she also carefully checked through manuscript and proofs. Mary Balfour, former chief executive of the AFV, gave us ample encouragement to initiate the project and to keep it going when it might otherwise have waned.

Two senior Melbourne physical therapists, Gabrielle Bortoluzzi (Box Hill Hospital) and Jill Exton (Children's Hospital), provided useful reactions and comments on the original manuscript, we are grateful to them and to several other members of the physical therapy profession who pointed us in the right direction. Deborah Merritt, of Hawaii Therapeutic Exercise, took an early interest in *Exercise Beats Arthritis* during her successful visit to Australia. Since then she has kept in touch with the book, offering constructive comments about the exercise. Deborah sees the book as being "helpful to many people, not just those with arthritis."

We are in debt to these and many other people for their help, encouragement, and ideas—not least to the Arthritis Foundation of Victoria itself.

About the Authors

Valerie Sayce trained as a physical therapist at the Lincoln Institute of Health Sciences in Victoria, Australia. At present she works at the Arthritis Foundation of Victoria as the physical activities educator. Her role there includes extensive involvement in development, training, and ongoing supervision of the AFV Water Exercise Recreation Program, the foundation's demonstration exercise team, Joint Action, and other education programs. She conducts regular land based and water based exercise classes for people with arthritis.

Her interest in exercise also includes experience in leading general aerobic exercise classes and exercise to music classes for pregnant women. She has wide experience in dance and movement, including ballet, ballroom dancing, folk dance, Tai Chi, and choreography for amateur theater.

Educated in Scotland, Ian Fraser has worked in education and in publishing for over twenty years. He has written two English textbooks and numerous other handbooks for teachers. His varied work experiences have included teaching, educational research, personnel, college administration, radio, and publishing. Exercise, he claims, is beating his osteoarthritis.

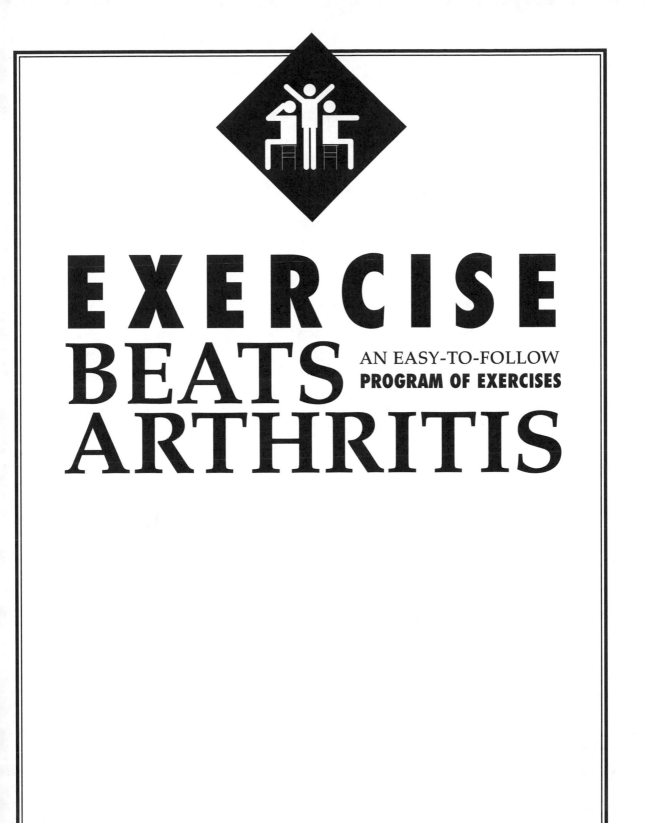

EXERCISE
BEATS
ARTHRITIS

AN EASY-TO-FOLLOW
PROGRAM OF EXERCISES

1

What Is Arthritis?

The word *arthritis* means literally inflammation of the joint. However, in general usage the term covers a multitude of problems affecting the joints, the muscles, and the connective tissues of the body. There are over one hundred different kinds of arthritis, but in this book we will discuss only the most common varieties.

If you are reading this book, you may have already been to your doctor who diagnosed your condition as arthritis, or maybe you just have a few aches and pains that you think might be arthritis.

What are the usual signs and symptoms of arthritis?

- Recurrent pain or tenderness in a joint
- Inability to move a joint normally
- Swelling, redness, or heat in one or more joints
- Joint stiffness when you wake up in the morning
- Unexplained loss of weight, fever, weakness, or fatigue, combined with joint pain

If any of these symptoms lasts for more than two weeks, you should see your doctor, who will be able to tell whether you have arthritis.

The various types of arthritis have specific effects on the different parts of the joint. You will understand more about your arthritis if you appreciate the function of the various structures within the normal joint.

1. *Bones:* Two bones meet to form the joint. The ends of the bones are smooth and shaped to fit into each other. It is the shape of the bones that determines the type of movement in a joint.

2. *Cartilage:* The surfaces of the bones within the joint are covered by cartilage. This is a smooth tough elastic substance that cushions and protects the ends of the bones.

3. *Joint capsule:* Completely surrounding the joint and holding everything together is the tough fibrous joint capsule.

4. *Synovial membrane:* Lining the inner surface of the joint capsule is a thin membrane called the synovial membrane.

5. *Synovial fluid:* The synovial membrane secretes a very important fluid with a consistency similar to egg-white. During movement, this synovial fluid is squeezed between the joint surfaces and acts as a lubricant to ensure the smooth function of the joint. It also provides nourishment to the joint cartilage.

6. *Ligaments:* These are short fibrous cords that reinforce the joint capsule and help maintain the stability of the joint.

7. *Muscles:* The joint is moved by the muscles that pass over it. Muscle tissue is elastic, so it can become shorter or longer. Movement of the joint occurs when the muscles contract.

8. *Tendons:* The muscles are usually attached to the bones by strong fibrous cords. These tendons are enclosed in a sheath that secretes synovial fluid to provide smooth movement.

9. *Bursa:* Near some joints there are small cushions between the bones and tendons or muscles. These bursae are small sacs lined with synovial membrane and filled with synovial fluid.

Rheumatoid Arthritis

What picture comes into your mind when you think about someone suffering with arthritis? Many people have the idea that arthritis is a painful and crippling disease resulting in unsightly joint deformities, and that anyone who has arthritis is severely restricted in what they are able to do. The disease that they have in mind is rheumatoid arthritis. It is true that in its most severe form, or when it is not well managed, rheumatoid arthritis can result in very painful and badly damaged joints—and much suffering. However, for most people with rheumatoid arthritis, it's quite possible to lead a fairly normal life.

Rheumatoid arthritis is a widespread disease. It affects about 3 percent of the

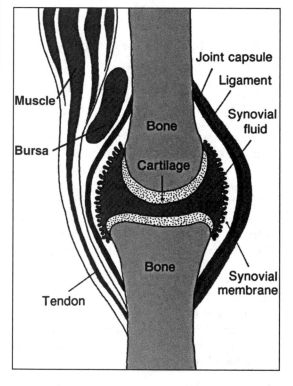

A normal joint

population, three-quarters of whom are women. Usually the disease begins in mid-life, but it can start at any age.

The course of the disease varies from person to person. In its mildest form, rheumatoid arthritis is an illness lasting only a few months and leaving no disability. Or it may come and go, with episodes of illness interspersed with periods of normal health. For most people, though, the disease progresses for a number of years with periods of flareup and remission. The rate of progress is very variable. Fortunately, in most cases the disease tends to burn itself out and after a time causes no further damage.

So what causes rheumatoid arthritis? What happens to your body? The exact cause is unknown, but it does involve the body's immune system, which normally protects you from disease. In rheumatoid arthritis, it

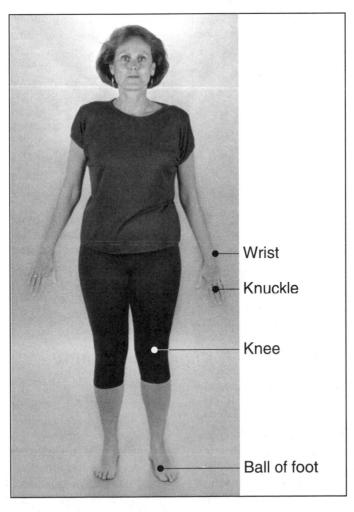

— Wrist

— Knuckle

— Knee

— Ball of foot

Common sites of rheumatiod arthritis

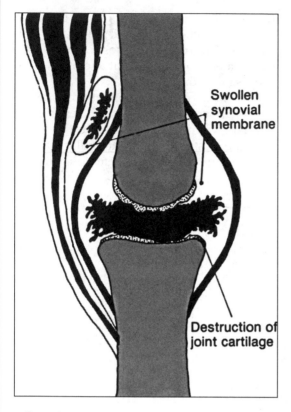

Effects of rheumatoid arthritis on a joint

appears that some causative factor triggers your immune system to react against your own tissues—in particular the joints. The result is that the synovial membrane lining the inside of the joint becomes inflamed and enlarged.

This makes the joint warm, swollen, and painful. The inflamed synovial tissue produces enzymes that are released into the joint. These cause more irritation and pain. Eventually the enzymes may eat away the structures inside the joint—cartilage, bone, ligaments—and this is what causes the permanent joint deformities.

Rheumatoid arthritis affects your whole body, not just your joints. It may cause inflammation in the muscles, tendons, lungs, skin, blood vessels, nerves, and eyes. Many people with rheumatoid arthritis feel generally tired and run down. Loss of appetite and weight is common. Some people have a slight fever.

Any joint can be affected by rheumatoid arthritis, but usually the same joints on both sides of the body are involved, most commonly the wrists, knuckles, knees, and the balls of the feet.

Treatment for rheumatoid arthritis reflects the variability of the disease and is really an individualized management program. It involves a combination of medication, rest, exercise, joint protection, and, in extreme circumstances, surgery. Common sense, a positive attitude, and understanding from others play a large part in a successful management program.

Exercise and Rheumatoid Arthritis

Rheumatoid arthritis requires a delicate balance of rest and activity. When your joints are hot, swollen, and painful, they need to be rested, although they should still be taken through their range of movement one or two times a day. At other times, regular exercise is essential in order to maintain the maximum function of joints and muscles.

This book gives you the opportunity to develop a suitable exercise program for your condition.

Osteoarthritis

How often do you hear someone complaining about an odd ache or pain and then dismissing it by saying, "I must be getting old"? As everyone gets older, their joints show some signs of degeneration, although for the majority of people this causes little or no problem. When this process starts to produce pain, it is known by a number of names: osteoarthritis, osteoarthrosis, OA, degenerative joint disease, cervical spondylosis (in the

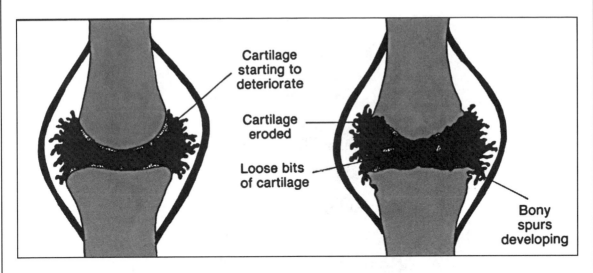

Cartilage starting to deteriorate

Cartilage eroded

Loose bits of cartilage

Bony spurs developing

Effects of osteoarthritis on a joint

neck), and lumbar spondylosis (in the lower back).

Osteoarthritis is a completely different condition from rheumatoid arthritis, although some people may have both. With osteoarthritis, only the joint itself is affected. Usually there is no inflammation. The main structure affected in osteoarthritis is the cartilage that covers the ends of the bones. It softens and becomes pitted and frayed, so movement is no longer smooth and easy. Cartilage has only a limited ability to heal itself since it does not have any blood supply.

With aging, the cartilage loses some of its resilience and is unable to absorb the same stresses as before. Gradually the cartilage is eroded, exposing the bone itself. In severe cases the destructive process can affect the underlying bony surfaces. Sometimes pieces of cartilage break off and float around in the joint. Moving an osteoarthritic joint can be very painful. Your body makes an effort to solve the problem by trying to increase the weight-bearing area of the joint. Bony spurs (called *osteophytes*) form in the places where the ligaments and joint capsule attach to the

bone. These osteophytes can themselves cause problems, particularly in the spine.

But not everyone develops osteoarthritis, so there must be factors other than age that contribute to the breakdown of the cartilage. It's possible that some people are born with less resilient cartilage, or that their joints do not fit together very well, or maybe they move incorrectly. Osteoarthritis is much more likely to develop in joints that have been injured in some way—say, through a fracture or dislocation, or if they have been subjected to too much load.

Contrary to what you might think, vigorous use of a joint does not necessarily lead to osteoarthritis. This is because it is through activity that the synovial fluid, which lubricates and nourishes the joint, is squeezed into the cartilage, and this seems to counteract any damage that may be happening.

Osteoarthritis can occur in any joint, but it is usually the joints under most stress that are commonly affected: hips, knees, neck, lower spine, the base of the big toe and thumb, and the end joints of

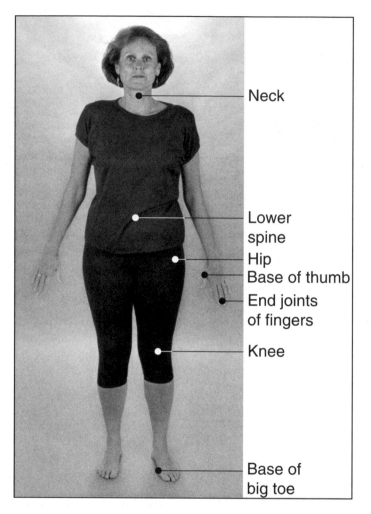

Neck

Lower spine

Hip

Base of thumb

End joints of fingers

Knee

Base of big toe

Common sites of osteoarthritis

the fingers. Some people, more often women, develop a bony thickening at the end finger joints.

Osteoarthritis is an ongoing degenerative condition, so treatment is aimed at relieving the symptoms and preventing further damage. Management involves a combination of exercise, rest, medication, weight control, comfort techniques, joint protection, and, only if absolutely necessary, surgery.

You can obtain a lot of relief by sticking faithfully to your treatment program.

Exercise and Osteoarthritis

Regular and appropriate exercise is probably the best way to get relief from your osteoarthritis. As we have already mentioned, the cartilage is nourished when you move your joints. So keeping active helps prevent further degeneration. Exercise will also strengthen the muscles around the joint, providing it with greater support.

This does not mean that you should undertake a strenuous exhausting exercise program, which will only cause more damage. Nor should you force yourself to exercise a very painful joint. Pain is a message from your body that something is wrong. You must take heed and rest the joint.

This book will help you to develop an exercise program suitable for your osteoarthritic joints.

Ankylosing Spondylitis

Ankylosing spondylitis is not a common form of arthritis, but it is one in which exercise plays a key part. The main feature of ankylosing spondylitis is stiffness of the spine, which can become completely rigid if the disease is not properly managed.

Ankylosing spondylitis is more prevalent among men than women, and usually affects younger people (15–25 years old). Often, however, symptoms are not recognized as ankylosing spondylitis until the person is a bit older.

Ankylosing spondylitis is different from other arthritic conditions in that it affects structures outside the joint, rather than inside. It starts with inflammation of the ends of the ligaments where they attach to the bone. The joint most commonly involved is the sacroiliac joint, the joint between the bottom of the spine and the pelvis.

The first symptom of ankylosing spondylitis is usually stiffness and pain in the lower back. The inflammation gradually spreads to the joints farther up the spine and may affect the attachment of the ribs to the spine. It may spread down to the hips, but only rarely are the other joints of the limbs involved.

The inflammation causes pain and stiffness, but this is not the end of the problem. After a while, bony outgrowths spread along the ligaments, forming a solid bridge between the two bones. Obviously, this means that the joint cannot move. The only benefit is that it is no longer painful. This fusion of the joints of the spine is what leads to the rigid "poker back" so characteristic of ankylosing spondylitis. However, good management helps prevent the disease from progressing this far. Most people are able to lead very active normal lives.

Exercise and Ankylosing Spondylitis

Exercise is the key to the successful management of ankylosing spondylitis. It is essential to keep the affected joints as mobile as possible. This involves a consistent active exercise program. Also, you need to be aware of your posture at all times–even when you are sleeping! If the bones are going to fuse together, you want them to be in the most functional position possible.

We have included a selection of exercises specifically for people with ankylosing spondylitis (see page 76). You will also find helpful exercises in the other sections—in particular breathing, neck, hips, and other back exercises.

Neck and Low Back Pain

Pain, tension, and discomfort in the neck and lower back are all too common. It is estimated that as many as four in every five people are significantly affected by low back pain at some time in their lives.

The spine is a complex structure of many different but interconnected parts. Any of these can be injured or strained, resulting in pain. Pain may be felt close to or

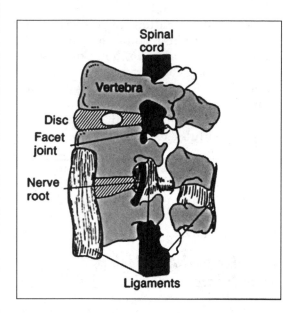

Structures of the spine

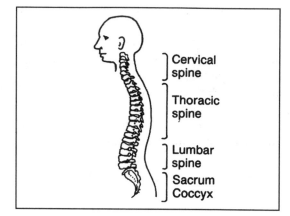

Normal spinal curves

some distance from the site of the problem. This can make it difficult to diagnose specific conditions.

The most common sites of pain are the neck and low back: these are also the most flexible and active sections of the spine. They are most vulnerable where they join the less flexible parts, such as the pelvis or upper back.

As well as producing pain in and around the spine, stimulation of any of the pain-sensitive structures deep in the back can cause more widespread pain and aching in other areas—notably the shoulders, arms, buttocks, and thighs. This is different from nerve root pain, such as sciatica, which is felt directly along the route of the nerve. Both, however, may be called referred pain.

Most back and neck pain is due to chronic strain or misuse of the facet joints, discs, and other supporting structures. Even when an injury results from a specific incident, it may have its origins in long-term stresses that show no obvious symptoms. The basis of this is often poor posture. The spine has a normal set of curves designed to align everything in the position of least stress. However, lack of exercise, sedentary work and leisure habits, increased weight, muscle imbalances, and tensions can all lead to changes in alignment. This changes the positioning and puts undue stress on the various spinal tissues. Eventually they protest that they are unable to do what is asked of them. Arthritis and disc degeneration can be a result of poor back care throughout life.

Exercise—both specific and general—plays a key role in preventing and overcoming neck and back pain. The exercises described in this book are appropriate for all forms of back and neck pain, not just that due to arthritis. Other strategies may include relaxation, back education, postural awareness, and, for acute episodes, possibly physiotherapy, rest, and medication.

Bursitis and Tendonitis

These are localized conditions in which there is inflammation of structures near a joint. They can be linked with arthritis, particularly rheumatoid arthritis, but more commonly they occur as separate conditions and have an obvious cause.

The fluid-filled cushion known as the bursa can become inflamed after an injury, after prolonged or repeated pressure, or through overuse. The most common sites of bursitis are around the shoulder, elbow, and knee. Water on the knee is a common phrase used to describe bursitis of the knee.

Inflammation of the tendons, which connect muscles to bone, may occur where they attach to the bone (tendonitis) or in the membranous sheath surrounding them (tenosynovitis). Common sites for these conditions are the shoulder, wrist, fingers, elbow, big toe, and heel. Everyone has heard of "tennis elbow." The cause is usually overuse, sudden stress, or unaccustomed use.

The symptoms associated with inflammation of these areas are pain, stiffness, swelling, and loss of use. Initially the best treatment is rest followed by gentle movement. Physical therapy and medication may be used if the problem persists.

Fibromyalgia Syndrome

Imagine the all-over pain, aching, stiffness, and exhaustion you experience with the flu. That is just how many people with fibromyalgia describe the way they feel most of the time! Properly known as fibromyalgia syndrome (FMS), it is a particular collection of symptoms, with the most common being extensive pain and aching throughout the body, persistent lack of energy, muscle stiffness, disturbed sleep, chronic headaches, irritable bowel, and other symptoms. You don't have to have all of these symptoms, but if you have a significant number, together with marked tenderness to pressure at 11 out of 18 specific "tender points" (see below), a diagnosis of fibromyalgia syndrome is likely. People of any age, including children and adoles-

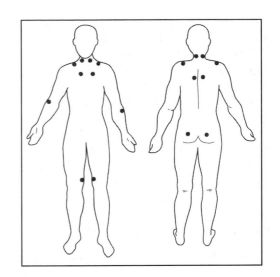

Diagnostic tender points defined by the American College of Rheumatology

cents, can develop fibromyalgia, but it is more common in women.

Fibromyalgia can often be very tricky to diagnose initially, because symptoms can fluctuate considerably and may be similar to some other rheumatic conditions. Sometimes it is a matter of ruling out everything else since all blood tests, X-rays, and other laboratory tests are normal. It's no wonder that many people with fibromyalgia sometimes get the feeling other people don't quite believe the significance of their problem and they can become very anxious and frustrated about what is happening to them.

It seems that in fibromyalgia the pain system has become overactive, resulting in a lower pain threshold. What this means is that your pain nerves are sensitive and much more ready to fire off and carry a pain message to your brain than they should be. At present we don't know what causes this change. It is possible for the pain system to return to normal. For some people, fibromyalgia seems to have been triggered by an injury, illness, or stressful event, although for others there is no obvious cause.

As with other forms of arthritis, treatment is largely a question of learning about the ways of managing the symptoms most effectively so that you can get on with your life. It is important to remember that, although the pain you are experiencing is "real," it is not due to tissue damage. Various pain and stress management strategies such as relaxation, meditation, heat, massage, counseling, and gentle exercise can be useful.

Exercise and Fibromyalgia

Exercise for fibromyalgia is essential so the problems of the condition are not further exacerbated by inactivity and lack of fitness. The best ways of exercising are stretches, rhythmic general movements, and aerobic conditioning that don't put too much strain on your body. People with fibromyalgia can be very sensitive to overexertion, so you need to start at a very low level of intensity and build up gradually and consistently. Shorter, more frequent periods of exercise are generally more effective. You are working too hard if you find you are exhausted or in a lot of pain after your exercise sessions. Cut back, but don't stop altogether.

Osteoporosis

Osteoporosis is a very common condition mainly affecting older women. The strength and density of the bones are reduced, thereby increasing the likelihood of having a fracture. Osteoporosis is not actually a form of arthritis, although the name is often confused with the common form of degenerative arthritis, osteoarthritis.

The bones of the skeleton are made of living tissue and constantly remodel themselves to adapt to the changing forces on them. Throughout life there is a continual turnover of bone cells, with new bone being formed and older bone being removed.

The structure of bone is that of a supporting framework strengthened by minerals, mainly calcium. The amount of calcium absorbed depends on three main factors. First, adequate calcium needs to be taken in so that it is available to perform its functions within the body as well as contributing to the strength of bones. Second, bone responds to how strong it needs to be. If forces acting on bone are increased, it responds by becoming stronger; similarly, a lack of stress results in weaker bone. Finally, calcium absorption largely depends on circulating female and male sex hormones—estrogen and testosterone.

The general pattern of bone mass variation with age is shown above. Rapid bone growth occurs during childhood and adolescence, a balance is maintained through early and mid adulthood, and an overall loss of bone occurs in later life. The most vital period for rapid bone growth is before and around the time of puberty, with peak bone mass (maximum amount of bone achieved) occurring about age 20. For women, the early years following menopause mean falling estrogen levels, and this accelerates bone loss. This is why older women are most susceptible to osteoporosis. The point at which the risk of sustaining a fracture is substantially increased is known as the fracture threshold. You can see how building up your peak bone mass in early life reaps its rewards later on since you are able to draw from a larger "bank" of bone.

Osteoporosis in itself is not painful, but a subsequent fracture certainly is and may have serious long-term consequences. Studies of people over 60 years of age indicate the disturbing statistic that about half of all women and nearly one-third of men will sustain a fracture due to osteoporosis.

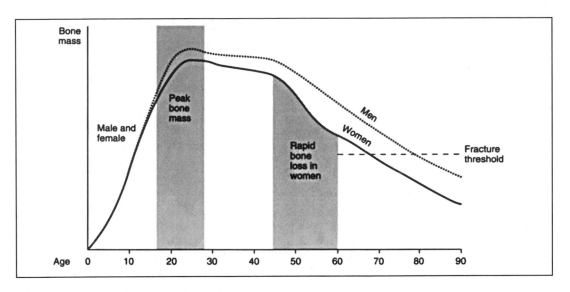

Changes in amount of bone with increasing age

Commonly, these osteoporotic fractures follow a relatively minor fall or knock and occur at the hip, wrist, upper arm, or ribs or as crush fractures in the spine.

Understanding Risk Factors

A combination of factors causes osteoporosis. Some you can do nothing about, but there are others in which you can make significant changes to help minimize bone loss.

- Genetic factors determine 60–80 percent of the peak bone mass level you will reach and the rate of bone you lose with advancing age. Lightly built females generally attain a lesser peak bone mass. It is small-framed women of Caucasian or Asian origin with a family history of osteoporosis who are most likely to develop osteoporosis.

- A woman's menstrual history relates to estrogen levels and has important consequences for bone mass. Delayed onset of puberty and early menopause, either natural or artificially induced, are both associated with lower bone mass, as are significant disruptions to the normal menstrual cycle due to excessive exercise or inadequate nutrition.

- Other chronic medical conditions (including rheumatoid arthritis) and certain medications (particularly corticosteroid drugs) may affect bone formation.

- Lifestyle factors can influence the amount of calcium you absorb into your bones, and these are what you can do something about. A low calcium intake or generally poor nutrition means there may not be enough calcium available for bone formation. A sedentary life-style at any age (childhood through to menopause) reduces the rate of bone formation. Also, calcium absorption is decreased by high alcohol consumption and by cigarette smoking.

Exercise and Osteoporosis

Bone formation is stimulated by the physical stress put on the skeleton through bearing the weight of the body and by muscles pulling strongly as they contract. At any age, regular exercise is essential in helping maintain bone strength. Choose activities that suit your level of ability.

- Weight-bearing exercise means the full force of gravity goes through the skeleton and includes such activities as walking, dancing, and low-impact aerobic classes. For those who do not have joint problems, greater stress is provided by the increased impact of jogging, climbing stairs and hills, high-impact aerobic classes, and more vigorous sports. Swimming, water exercise, and cycling are not classed as weight-bearing although they have other important health benefits.
- High resistance weight-training also encourages bone formation. For help in developing a safe and effective gymnasium program, consult a qualified weight-training instructor.

Regular exercise can protect your bones in other ways. By improving balance, coordination, flexibility, muscle strength, and posture, exercise helps reduce your risk of having a fall that may result in a fracture.

And an appeal to parents and grandparents of young girls: Whenever possible, encourage adolescent girls to participate in some form of vigorous weight-bearing activity to help build up their peak bone mass.

Other Considerations in Prevention and Management

- An adequate intake of calcium throughout life is vital. The recommended daily intake is 1000 milligrams (mg) for adolescent girls (12–15 years) and post-menopausal women, 1100–1200 mg for women who are pregnant or breastfeeding, and 800 mg for adult women (19–54 years). The most readily absorbed source of calcium is dairy products (milk, yogurt, cheese) with low-fat varieties having just as much calcium as full-cream. Other sources of calcium include canned fish (with bones), dark green leafy vegetables, and dried beans. Calcium supplements are available if you do not have enough calcium in your diet. Talk to your doctor about whether this is necessary and which to get.
- Bone density measurement can detect bone loss and is helpful in the diagnosis and management of osteoporosis. The most accurate method of bone density measurement is a DEXA scan (dual energy X-ray absorptiometry).
- Hormone replacement therapy (HRT) following menopause may be very effective in preventing the anticipated rapid bone loss. For some women there are concerns about taking HRT, so it is best to discuss your own situation with your doctor.
- Other medications are now becoming available that can help restore or slow down some of the bone loss. If you have established osteoporosis, you can discuss the options available with your doctor.

• Obviously you are more likely to have a fracture if you fall. Along with regular exercise you can help prevent falls by being aware of dangerous situations at home and in public places. At home, check for slippery floors and pathways, loose mats, poor lighting at night, and cluttered rooms. Install handrails on stairs and in the bathroom and toilet. Other important safety measures include using a walking aid if you need it, having your eyesight checked regularly, and consulting your doctor or pharmacist about any medications that may be affecting your balance.

Let's Find Out About

Diet

Some of the most common questions asked by people with arthritis relate to diet: "Should I eat more of this? Should I avoid these foods? Will it help if I take this supplement?" Often, in magazine articles, people are said to be miraculously cured of their arthritis by following a particular diet. But the answer may not be that simple. There are a number of reasons why it is difficult to determine what caused the person's improvement.

First, don't lose sight of the fact that arthritis is not a single disease, but a name that covers a wide range of very different conditions. This means that what helps one form of arthritis may not work for another.

Second, one of the characteristics of arthritis—particularly rheumatoid arthritis—is that it comes and goes. How can we

be certain that a particular remission is due to a change of diet?

Also, your weight affects the amount of strain you put on your joints. Most diets, if followed strictly, will result in some loss of weight even if they are not designed to do so.

The final point is that your mental attitude has a great effect on your perception of pain and your ability to cope with it. Enthusiastically embarking on a new diet can be a very positive step towards helping yourself—a move that challenges the influence your arthritis has on you.

All this does not mean that diet is not a significant factor in managing your arthritis. It is. But there are no scientific studies that prove that specific foods are directly related to arthritis. The only exception is gout. People who have had an attack of gout can usually control further episodes by taking certain dietary precautions.

How then can diet help your arthritis? There are two main ways:

- A nutritious well-balanced diet is good for everyone.

- Being overweight adds to the problems of arthritic joints.

By eating a nourishing diet, you can be sure that your body is receiving all the necessary nutrients to give you energy, keep you healthy, and repair damaged tissues.

People who are overweight put more strain on their joints—especially those of the back and lower limbs. They are generally less active, too, and more prone to other illnesses such as heart and circulatory conditions and diabetes.

The Food Guide Pyramid is an excellent guide to good nutrition and a balanced diet. It offers us a visual representation of the Dietary Guidelines. It emphasizes complex carbohydrates, fruits, and vegetables as the source of calories, hence their position at the "base." The number of servings needed depends on one's calorie needs, which vary with age, sex, physical condition, and activity levels.

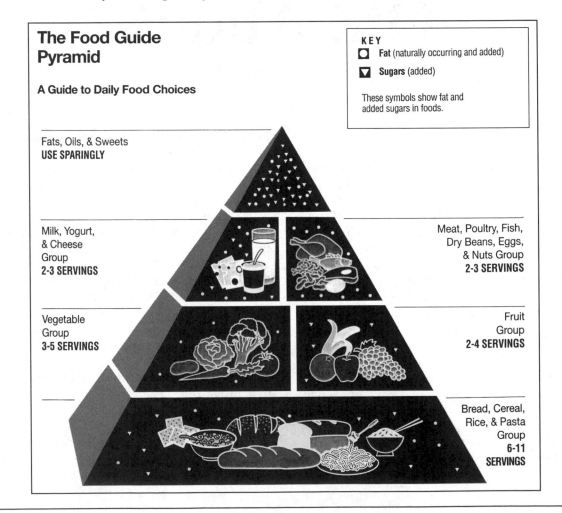

The Food Guide Pyramid

A Guide to Daily Food Choices

KEY
☐ **Fat** (naturally occurring and added)
▼ **Sugars** (added)

These symbols show fat and added sugars in foods.

Fats, Oils, & Sweets
USE SPARINGLY

Milk, Yogurt, & Cheese Group
2-3 SERVINGS

Meat, Poultry, Fish, Dry Beans, Eggs, & Nuts Group
2-3 SERVINGS

Vegetable Group
3-5 SERVINGS

Fruit Group
2-4 SERVINGS

Bread, Cereal, Rice, & Pasta Group
6-11 SERVINGS

Try to avoid foods that contain preservatives and other chemical additives. Limit your salt intake, as well as your consumption of alcohol and caffeine. The dangers to your health of cigarette smoking are now well known.

If you are overweight, you need to consume fewer calories than you use up. Exercise and increased activity will certainly help. As far as diet is concerned, concentrate on the lower parts of the pyramid. Don't try to lose too much weight too quickly. Weight that comes off slowly is more likely to stay off.

Some people with rheumatoid arthritis have the problem of being underweight. It's a mistake to try to gain weight by eating sweet rich fatty foods. These supply calories but not a lot of nutrients. Concentrate instead toward the middle of the pyramid, which contains foods that are both nourishing and fairly high in calories.

Mental Attitude

Your attitude about your arthritis and your expectations about it are two major factors in determining how much effect arthritis has on your life. Anxiety, pain, and fatigue are all associated with feelings of depression. It's very easy to let yourself become more and more miserable and less able to cope with your daily activities.

There are many ways to help lift yourself out of this cycle, but the first big step is for you to *decide that you want to help yourself.* Friends and relatives, church and community groups, counselors, your doctor, and other health professionals can all give you guidance, but *you* are the one who is ultimately in control of your own life and your attitude toward it. Once you have a positive focus, you will probably find that your arthritis no longer bothers you to the same degree.

Stress

Have you found that your arthritis is worse when you are under physical or emotional stress? This is very common. It seems that when we try to push ourselves too far our bodies start to give way at their weakest links. For people with arthritis, this is their joints.

Sometimes the onset of rheumatoid arthritis coincides with a period of severe stress in a person's life. This is not to say that stress causes arthritis, but it is possibly a contributing factor. And once you have arthritis, it is certainly affected by stress. Medicine today is acknowledging the close relationship between our minds and our bodies.

Of course, it is impossible to rid yourself of all stress in your life. The unexpected can always happen. But you can try to eliminate many unnecessary day-to-day stresses by:

- Planning ahead
- Being realistic about time and your capabilities
- Assessing your priorities
- Sharing responsibilities
- Asking for help
- Practicing relaxation

Visiting the Doctor

Aches, pains, and minor injuries of our joints are very common. After giving us a few days of discomfort, they usually go away of their own accord. People often wonder whether they should go to their doctor or not. In general, there is not a lot the doctor can do to help these minor nonspecific ailments. Probably, you will be advised to rest the part and take some mild form of pain relief.

However, you do not have to suffer in silence in the mistaken belief that nothing can be done or doctors don't want to listen. If you have any one or more of the following symptoms for more than two weeks, then you should make an appointment to see your doctor:

- Persistent or recurrent pain in any joint
- Swelling in one or more joints
- Redness and warmth in a joint
- Early-morning stiffness
- Inability to move a joint normally
- Unexplained weight loss, fever, or weakness, combined with joint pain.

When you go to your doctor, he or she will take your history and give you a physical examination. This may be all that is needed to establish a diagnosis of arthritis. Sometimes the doctor will want a bit more information in order to confirm the diagnosis or to rule out other possibilities. The most usual investigations are blood tests and X-rays.

Initially, of course, you would start with your local doctor. But if your arthritis is not responding well to treatment or if there is a specific point of concern, you or your doctor may suggest that you see a rheumatologist, a doctor who specializes in rheumatic and arthritic conditions.

However, your main contact will still be with your doctor, so it is important that you have someone with whom you feel comfortable. Both you and your doctor must have respect for each other. The doctor has theoretical knowledge of and experience with arthritis and its treatment, but you are the only one who knows how your body feels. Find a doctor with whom you can build up a good line of communication, and you are much more likely to get results.

You can help your doctor, too, by preparing the questions you wish to ask and by making sure you understand any advice or instructions given. Don't be embarrassed about asking for further explanations. Your doctor will also be interested in hearing about anything you have found helpful, as your experience can then be passed on to other people. Arthritis is a very individual disease and so needs a personally tailored treatment program. It needs good cooperation between doctor and patient to achieve the most satisfactory results.

Medication

When you first went to a doctor about your arthritis, you were probably given a prescription for some pills or tablets. It's true that medication has a place in the treatment of arthritis, but sometimes both patients and doctors rely too heavily on drugs as the only means of controlling arthritis. All drugs have side effects, and some people do not tolerate certain drugs as well as others.

When considering drug therapy, it is important to realize the difference between rheumatoid arthritis and osteoarthritis. With rheumatoid arthritis the main problem is inflammation. A reduction in this will ease the pain. To be effective, medication for the control of inflammation must be ongoing. With osteoarthritis there is usually no inflammation. The main concern is just pain! Therefore the medication is related to the amount of pain you are experiencing.

There is one important word of caution about drugs. Be sure to consult fully with your doctor about your medication. Don't stop taking a drug or change the dosage without letting your doctor know. Also make sure you understand and follow the dosage instructions. You must remember that you are dealing with potentially damaging substances.

Aspirin: Aspirin is a common drug used for arthritis. It has two main beneficial effects: it relieves pain and it reduces inflammation. Pain relief is obviously important for people with arthritis, but it is aspirin's anti-inflammatory properties that make it (and its related drugs) so useful in dealing with rheumatoid arthritis. The most common side effect of aspirin is irritation of the lining of the stomach.

Nonsteroidal anti-inflammatory drugs: This is a diverse group of drugs that may be classed as aspirin substitutes. Their main action is to reduce inflammation, so they are particularly useful for rheumatoid arthritis. They are derived from different chemical families, so particular drugs are more suited to certain individuals. It may mean a bit of trial and error to discover which is the most suitable drug for your condition. They do not seem to have the same side effects as aspirin, but because they are newer, we cannot be sure of the hazards of long-term use.

Antimalarials: The drugs developed for the control of malaria have also been found to help reduce the inflammation of rheumatoid arthritis. They may be used with other drugs and are usually very well tolerated without serious side effects.

Remittive agents: Everyone has probably heard of gold injections for rheumatoid arthritis. Gold and penicillamine are two different drugs with similar effects on joint inflammation. They can produce a dramatic reduction in symptoms and may even result in a remission. However, they do have potentially hazardous side effects and must be used with discretion and be carefully monitored.

Corticosteroids: When it was first developed, cortisone was thought to be a wonder drug for rheumatoid arthritis. Since then, some serious side effects from long-term use have been found. Cortisone is still useful as a treatment for rheumatoid arthritis, but it should be used with great caution and be strictly supervised. Cortisone injections are sometimes given into a particularly troublesome joint. They may give excellent relief lasting for months, but this is not always the case. Although the injections do not have the same side effects as taking the drug orally, they must still be used discriminately.

Immunosuppressives: These are very powerful and dangerous drugs that work by suppressing the body's immune system. In all except the most serious forms of arthritis, the risks of side effects outweigh any potential benefits.

Other Health Professionals

Part of your treatment program may include physical therapy. A physical therapist knows a lot about how the muscles and joints of your body work. Your physical therapy treatment may include an individualized exercise program, hydrotherapy, heat treatment, appropriate splinting, advice on suitable footwear, instruction on the use of walking aids, education in the best ways to use your body and protect your joints, and how to balance your daily activities.

Occupational therapists are concerned with helping you to function better and more independently in your daily activities. This may include various aids and devices and suggestions on how to adapt your home so you can do as much as possible for yourself with the least amount of strain on your joints.

Medication is often a cause of concern. Do remember that your local pharmacist is often a good source of information on how drugs work and can help you understand your doctor's instructions.

Surgery

There are times when a joint is so badly affected and causes so much pain that the only resort is to surgery. You have probably heard or know of people with artificial hips. It is certainly true that these have been a great success in restoring function and relieving the pain of a severely arthritic hip.

Surgery needs to be approached with caution and careful consideration. It is not always a success, although for many people it has given them a new lease on life. If you are thinking of surgery, then it's wise to consult more than one surgeon. Find someone well experienced in the type of operation you require. It is also a good idea to talk to someone who has had the operation you are considering.

Of course, not all arthritic conditions are suitable for surgery. In general, surgery is most useful when the problem is localized to one joint and is most successful for the larger joints such as the hip and knee. Joint replacement has been a great help to people with severe arthritis in the hip or knee. Replacements of other joints (shoulder, ankle, elbow, fingers) are being worked on and are becoming more successful.

Comfort Techniques

You have probably found that it is the continual day-to-day pain and discomfort of arthritis that is most upsetting. To cope better with this, you can build up a store of techniques that you know will help to make you more comfortable. This is a big part of "living with arthritis." These comfort techniques can make quite a difference to the amount of pain relief you require from drugs:

- Usually warmth helps to ease the pain. Wrap a towel around a hot water bottle or a hot pack (available from pharmacists) and cover the painful area. *Caution: this should feel warm, not hot. Be especially careful if you have sensitive skin.*
- Many heat rubs are available that you can massage into your joints. *Caution: never use these with other forms of direct heat, and be careful if you have sensitive skin.*
- Soak your hands or feet in a basin of warm water or your whole body in a warm bath.
- A gentle soothing massage from friendly hands is very comforting.
- During the day, thermal underwear, gloves, and scarves help keep you warm; and when you are considering what to wear, remember that wool retains warmth better than synthetic materials.
- Electric blankets, flannel sheets, and down conforters help keep you warm through the night.
- Try wearing socks, gloves, leg warmers, and knee or elbow socks to bed to retain the warmth in your joints.
- If possible, warm the room before you get up.

Do not apply heat to a hot swollen joint—it won't help. If at any time heat is making your joint feel worse instead of more comfortable, then don't continue with it.

Joint Protection

If you have arthritis, you need to be constantly aware of how much stress you are putting on your joints. Your aim is to prevent undue strain on your joints, so as to minimize your pain and keep them working for as long as possible. You need to balance activity with rest. Do not use your joints unnecessarily if they are painful—and try to avoid using them at all if they are hot and swollen.

Joint protection means using your joints wisely. Make sure that you lift, stand and move in a way that puts least stress on your joints (refer to pages 128–131). Use the larger, stronger joints to do the work, and try to distribute any load you are carrying over several joints. Think before you try to do a particular task. You are very likely to discover an easier, less stressful way of doing it.

Various aids and devices have been developed to take the strain off tender joints. Do you know that you can obtain gadgets that help you to put on stockings and socks, comb your hair, open cans and jars, turn on taps, hold pens and cutlery, pick things up off the floor, do the gardening, pull out plugs from the wall, and many other daily activities? An occupational therapist or the Arthritis Foundation can give you advice on where to obtain these useful devices.

The Weather

Do you believe you can predict the weather with at least as much accuracy as the weather bureau? Many people find that their arthritis seems to be aggravated by an impending change of weather—that is, when the barometric pressure is rising or falling.

As far as general climate is concerned, it seems that dampness and humidity have the most disturbing effects, so both cold and wet days or hot and humid ones can be very uncomfortable. Windy changeable weather is also not well tolerated. Although the climate does not seem to be related to the prevalence of arthritis, the day-to-day weather often has some bearing on the amount of pain experienced in arthritic joints.

It is worth noting whether the weather seems to affect your arthritis, because it may account for a particularly bad day and at least you know it will pass!

3

Your Exercise Program

Why Exercise?

Current medical and scientific evidence shows that exercise is one of the most useful and direct ways of minimizing the pain and limitations of arthritis. In certain circumstances it may even reverse some arthritic changes. It is now recognized that some symptoms usually associated with arthritis may simply be due to lack of exercise. A period of inactivity for anyone soon contributes to joint deterioration, muscle stiffness and weakness, fatigue, poor appetite, low pain threshold, osteoporosis, and depression. Many of these symptoms occur in a person with arthritis. So if you have arthritis and you do not do much exercise, it is hard to say whether your symptoms are due to arthritis, or inactivity, or a combination of the two.

You can understand, then, why there has been an upsurge of interest in improving fitness. The many physical and psychological benefits of exercise are well recognized, so by doing something for your arthritis you may well improve your overall health and well-being.

Exercise can contribute to:

- more efficient heart and lung function
- reduction in blood pressure
- weight control
- improvement in posture, balance, and coordination
- increased strength of muscles and bones
- joint nourishment and lubrication

- greater joint mobility and function
- relief of muscle tension, stress, and anxiety
- improved sleep patterns
- greater mental alertness
- development of a positive attitude and better self-image

Types of Exercise

To get all these benefits, you will need to include different activities in your exercise program. There are three categories of exercise, according to whether they aim to improve flexibility, strength, or aerobic conditioning. Often a particular exercise will work on more than one area. All three types are important in planning an overall fitness plan that will benefit your whole body, including your arthritis.

Flexibility exercises move the joints and muscles through their full range of motion and gradually increase how far they can move and the ease at which they move. As a joint becomes more mobile, it is able to function more effectively with less pain, and there is a reduced risk of overstraining. These exercises also help to relieve the early-morning stiffness often associated with arthritis. Exercises to make you more flexible involve a large range of movement, but they should not require too much effort. Only at the ends of the movement range, where stiffness is greatest, is gentle pressure required.

Strengthening exercises increase the strength of the muscles that move, support and protect the joints. Muscle wasting and weakness often accompany painful joints, making them less able to absorb shock and more likely to tire. You can feel your muscles contracting and working strongly as you do these exercises.

Flexibility and strengthening exercises complement each other, and both should be done as part of your exercise program. An arthritic joint will function better if it has good support, full range of movement, and adequate muscle strength. The exercises in this book often include flexibility and strengthening in varying proportions, so you get two benefits for the price of one!

Aerobic or endurance exercises enhance your overall fitness level by stimulating your lungs and cardiovascular system. They help reduce weight by increasing your body's energy consumption and often act as energizers by promoting a sense of well-being. This important form of exercise is often neglected by people with arthritis, but the general health benefits are a big plus in coping with arthritis. Aerobic exercise will be discussed in detail later in the book (see page 115).

Exercise with Care

For your exercise program, you need to choose activities that do not put too much strain on your joints. You can well imagine that weight lifting is not the best exercise for an arthritic shoulder, nor is downhill skiing sensible if you have osteoarthritis in your knee. Contact sports are obviously unwise for people with arthritis. Still, do not despair: there are plenty of other sports and activities less likely to cause damage, such as tennis, golf, folk dancing, and swimming. Use your common sense and choose something that does not put too much stress on your affected joints. And be sure to take it easy when your joints are painful.

If you are doing anything that involves running or walking, wear good supportive jogging shoes—the kind that will absorb some of the shock and so protect your joints.

Swimming and other water activities are excellent for people with arthritis. The buoyancy of water relieves much of the weight from your joints. Many of the exercises in this book can be done in the water.

At first, it is difficult to know how much exercise to do or when you have done too much. But experience is a great teacher. A good rule to go by is that, if you experience *exercise-induced pain for more than two hours* after the exercise period, then you have overdone it. Next time do a little less. Some muscle soreness is quite normal after unaccustomed exercise. But you want to avoid the pain caused by your joints being irritated by too much exercise.

Pain, as we have said, is a warning you are causing damage to your body. The cliché that "the more it hurts, the more good it's doing" is simply not true.

The exercises described in this book are all free active movements without assistance or resistance from any outside force. They have been developed for people with mild to moderate arthritis. If you practice them regularly, you will strengthen your muscles and stretch your joints. The exercises won't put excess strain on your joints, although some people will not be able to do all the exercises. *Do not do any exercise that causes you pain.* Do, however, make a gentle attempt at the same exercise a week or so later. There may be a pleasant surprise in store for you. Your stronger muscles and joints may now allow you to do the exercise more easily.

There is one time when you should avoid exercising a joint—namely, when it is severely inflamed. The common term for this is that the joint is *hot* or *flared up.* This is particularly relevant for those with rheumatoid arthritis or other inflammatory forms of arthritis. In this condition, the joint is very painful to move anyway. Too much movement could worsen the inflammation and cause damage to the joint. It needs to be rested. However, gentle movement through its relatively pain-free range is recommended to prevent stiffness.

Who Should Exercise

The exercise program described in this book has been developed to suit long-term mild to moderate arthritic problems. This means that your arthritis has been around for a while, but you don't have marked joint deformities, and in general your arthritis does not greatly hinder you in your normal daily activities.

The program is still suitable if you have had a hip or knee replacement, provided you take note of the precautions mentioned with particular exercises. It is possible to adapt many of the exercises if you have more severe arthritis, but be sure to consult a physical therapist or your doctor first. If you have any questions about the suitability of a particular exercise, you should seek professional help.

What to Exercise

No doubt certain parts of your body give you more problems than others, and of course the bothersome part may change from time to time. When you start your program, concentrate on one or two areas at a time, rather than trying to fix everything at once. You may even be surprised to find that the improvement in one part is reflected throughout the rest of your body.

It is worthwhile going through some exercises for all parts of the body in the course of the week, even if you have arthritis in just one joint. There are two very good reasons for doing this. First, some forms of arthritis affect different parts of the body, at various times. You can stay one step ahead by regularly exercising *all* your joints. The other point is that all the joints of your body are actually linked together, so that a problem in one part will affect the load placed on the joint next to it and so on through your body. Your joints do not work as isolated units but rather as moving parts of a whole functional body. Exercising all your joints will give support to present problem areas and will help prevent future problems.

When to Exercise

Any time of day will do. Only you can choose the most suitable time. But here are some general guidelines and considerations that may help you:

- You need an uninterrupted 15–30 minutes per day.
- Choose a time of day when you are feeling near your best—not when you are tired or in pain.
- If you are taking medication, try to exercise about half an hour after your regular dose—when it is at its most effective.
- Don't exercise on a full stomach.
- Break your exercise session into more than one period, if you wish.

Where to Exercise

The room you use needs to be well ventilated and neither too cold nor too warm. Make sure you have enough space in which to stretch out. In warm sunny weather, think about going into the fresh air for your exercise session.

For the floor exercises, you might be more comfortable lying on a mat or piece of foam. If you cannot get down onto the floor, lie on the bed if it has a firm base, although a bed is not as satisfactory as the floor. For the exercises done sitting, use a firm-based chair or stool that is the right height to support your thighs with your feet flat on the floor.

What to Wear

The clothes you wear for exercising should allow you to move freely and keep you warm. Just be careful not to cool off too quickly after your exercise period. Put back on any clothes you removed as you warmed up through your exercise session.

If you have problems with your feet, wear flat, comfortable, well-fitting, supportive shoes—particularly for any exercises done while standing. Avoid slip-on footwear and any that does not have a closed-in heel. Otherwise, for the flexibility and strengthening exercises, you can choose either to wear suitable shoes or to exercise in bare feet—whichever you find most comfortable.

Before You Exercise

If you are feeling very stiff and sore, you could perhaps spend 15–20 minutes warming your joints with one of the comfort techniques described on page 20. The relief from pain and the extra blood flow in the area will allow you to move more easily. *Do not take extra medication* to mask the pain you might feel during exercises. After all, pain is an indication you might be causing damage.

How to Exercise

To get the greatest benefit from exercises, give yourself enough time to do them properly. If your time is limited, it is better to do fewer exercises well, rather than rushing through a greater number.

When you are performing a particular exercise, concentrate on the part of your body that is being exercised. Feel how your joint is moving and which muscles are working. This awareness will help you to coordinate the movement. Make your movements smooth, rhythmic, and at an easy pace. You may overstrain your joints if you try to move too vigorously.

We have suggested that you start with 2–4 repetitions of each exercise. If you have no painful aftereffects, gradually build this up to 5–6 at the rate of one extra repetition per week. If the joint becomes tender, then decrease the number of repetitions. Refrain from exercising a joint that has flared up and become hot, swollen, and painful. Just move the joint very gently through its range of movement twice a day.

And don't forget to keep breathing as you exercise! Your muscles need oxygen in order to work. Sometimes you can find yourself holding your breath unintentionally, particularly with difficult or uncomfortable movements. Coordinating movement with your breathing can help you exercise. Breathe in with one part of the movement, then breathe out with another. In general, think of breathing in (expanding your chest) with opening or lifting movements, and breathing out (deflating your chest) with closing movements.

Some people find their exercise sessions much more enjoyable if they move to music. This is a good idea, but a word of caution about your choice of music. If it has a strong fast beat, you may be tempted to keep in time and so move your joints too vigorously. Slow gentle background music or pleasant easy-listening music is best.

Remember these important points:

- Consult your doctor or physical therapist if you have severe arthritis or are unsure about the suitability of an exercise.
- Do not continue with an exercise that is causing severe pain or discomfort.
- If you experience exercise-induced pain for more than about two hours, do less next time.
- Rest an inflamed joint.

After You Exercise

The time following an exercise period is an ideal time to practice relaxation. Muscles and joints are then ready to release their tension. If you do not have time for a relaxation session, then just allow yourself to ease gradually back into your daily activities. Even though the exercises did not seem so energetic at the time, you could find that you are quite tired afterward.

Also, be aware of your pain level after your exercise session. You have done too much if you have exercise-induced pain for more than two hours.

Planning Your Exercise Program

Developing a balanced exercise program that fits in well with your daily routine may take a bit of time. The first step is to realize that exercise must become one of your priority activities since it is going to help you lead a more enjoyable and satisfying life. An exercise program will only work and be safe if it is done regularly and consistently. This will take some planning and a good deal of commitment.

First, think about what you are doing through the days of the coming week. When and where can you fit in your exercise sessions? Now, make a definite commitment to a certain number of sessions over the week at specific times during the day. You could relate these sessions to something that is already part of your daily routine. Be realistic. Aim for 3–5 sessions a week rather than an optimistic session every day. If you do exercise more often than you planned, congratulate yourself heartily!

A good way to make your commitment work is to make a written contract with yourself. For instance:

During the next week I will do the following exercise activities.

Example	Your contract
Monday	_____
20 minutes of exercises from book before	_____
breakfast after morning shower.	_____
10 minutes of relaxation after lunch.	_____
Wednesday	_____
Water exercise class.	_____
20-minute walk after lunch.	_____
Visit friend nearby.	_____
Maybe friend will come on walk.	_____
Thursday or Friday	_____
Same as Monday.	_____
Saturday or Sunday	_____
20-minute walk with someone in family.	_____
Will arrange tonight.	_____
15 minutes of relaxation each day.	_____

Now you must decide which exercise activity to do for each exercise session. You certainly do not need to do exactly the same exercises every day.

The exercises in this book have been divided into sections:

Morning Wake-Up   page 33

Warm-Up   page 43

Neck   page 49

Arms   page 53

Hands   page 59

Back   page 65

Hips   page 79

Knees   page 85

Feet   page 91

Cool-Down   page 97

Water Exercise   page 103

Aerobic Exercise   page 115

Relaxation   page 119

Each section includes a short introduction before the exercises are described. This gives some background to what you might expect from arthritis in that area, the purpose of the exercises, and any precautions you need to take.

When you do an exercise for the first time, read through all the instructions before you start to move. Study the pictures and directions so you understand the exercise properly.

The *Key Exercises* have been chosen as the ones which are generally the most important for that body part. Through your own experience or by following the advice of your physical therapist or doctor, you may choose your own Key Exercises. Key Exercises are marked by a star (*).

The choices may seem overwhelming at first, but they have all been included so that you can find something that particularly suits you. Here are some guidelines to help you set up your individual exercise program.

1. Doing something is far better than doing nothing. So don't worry about having to make the perfect choice the first time. Experience will guide you in developing a program that is specifically yours.

2. Choose exercises and activities that appeal to you. Don't be afraid to try something different.

3. The length of your exercise session may vary considerably depending on your available time. Some days you will only have 15 minutes, other days you can devote an hour or more to exercise, or you may prefer two or three shorter sessions through the day.

4. Determine your priority joints. These are the ones giving you the most trouble at present. Start by choosing some exercises that concentrate on these.

5. Try to exercise all parts of the body over a one-week period. This can be done by including at least the Key Exercises for each body area.

6. Aerobic exercise is most effective if done three times per week. You can use some of the other exercises as a warm-up for your aerobic activity.

7. If you are stiff in the morning, always try to include the Morning Wake-Up. It will help you for the rest of the day. Try doing the same routine in bed at night and see if it makes any difference in how you feel the next morning.

8. Keep an exercise diary like the one shown below. This way you can note your progress and any problems. It is surprisingly effective in helping to make exercise a habit in your life. Keep the diary somewhere obvious and each day write in what you have done. You can also use it to plan your activities for the following days.

Maintaining Motivation

Starting is almost easy compared to keeping going. Hopefully, the benefits of regular exercise will soon be obvious and this will inspire you to continue. However, there are always times when progress is slow or you even feel you are going backward. This is a good time to reassess your exercise program and see if there are ways to give it a spark.

• Beware of overenthusiasm. It usually results in the activity being short-lived. If you have not done much exercise re-

Day	Exercise details	Aerobic exercise	Relaxation	Comments
Monday	Morning wake up. Warm up. Key ex.- Neck, Arms, Back. All hip exercises	20 min. walk	15 mins.	Increased pain at night. Very tired. Too much, I think!
Tuesday	morning wake up. warm up. Key ex. – Hip cool Down.		15 mins	Still tired. Pain less.
Wednesday	morning wake up. Did video exercise routine with friend.	10 min. walk to and from friend's house.	10 mins. (from video)	Enjoyed doing ex. with friend. We plan to do so each wednesday. Feeling very tired.
Thursday	morning wake up. Rest	Today	20 mins.	Felt very tired and in pain this morning. Need to slow down.
Friday	Water exercise class.		30mins.	Feeling much better after class.
Saturday	morning wake up. went with friend to local pool and did water ex. from book and had a swim.			No pain.
Sunday	Morning wake up. Rest	Today	30 mins.	Feeling good and not as stiff.

cently, a sudden burst of activity is likely to do more harm than good. Then you are left feeling that all your good intentions have been wasted. Be sensible. Follow the guidelines. Gradually increase the amount of exercise you do.

- Be realistic about your expectations. Your arthritis has probably been developing over many years, so is it reasonable to expect it to go away dramatically overnight? It is more likely you will barely notice the subtle improvements until you suddenly realize you are doing something you could not do before.

- For the first week or two, despite all precautions, your general pain level may increase as your joints and muscles move in unaccustomed ways. If you continue doing the exercises regularly and carefully, this should soon pass. If it does not, or if the pain is severe, stop and go to your doctor for advice.

- What about building your exercise time into your daily routine by connecting it with other activities? That way you will not run out of time or conveniently "forget." For instance, plan to do some exercise after your morning shower or before lunch.

- Vary your activities over time. As you become fitter, you will be able to do more each day.

- Set realistic targets. There will be days when you do not feel like doing anything, circumstances suddenly change, or something unexpected happens. Be kind to yourself by building some rest days into your program. This means you are more likely to achieve your goals. If you aim too high initially, you are just setting yourself up for increased pain and ultimate failure.

- Be honest with yourself about why you missed a session you had planned to do. Sometimes this is unavoidable, but often you can change the circumstances by asking for other people's cooperation or by reassessing your priorities. You can motivate yourself by arranging to follow your exercise session with a reward (not a piece of chocolate cake, though!). For instance, plan to telephone your friend after, rather than before, your exercise session.

- Setbacks and feelings of not getting anywhere are almost inevitable. Don't let them worry you. Instead, look back to when you first started, and you will realize your overall progress.

- Don't stop exercising when you start to improve. It is all right to have an occasional day off, but once you get out of the habit of regular exercise it is hard to crank up again. And, worst of all, you will soon find that all your hard-won improvements start to slip away.

- Feeling down is commonly associated with fatigue and lack of motivation. The best remedy is making contact with someone else and doing something together. Of course, chronic fatigue may be a symptom of some other condition. Check with your doctor if you are concerned.

- Plan to do some exercise sessions with a friend or group. This gives you the opportunity to discuss your exercise plans, report on progress, and use someone else's enthusiasm to rekindle your own flame.

- Contract with a friend or someone in your family. Say what you are going to do over the next week; be specific about time and place. Make this goal something that you can accomplish fairly easily but, at the same time, does require you to make some changes in your behavior. For instance, you say, "I will take a walk to visit a friend twice during the next week." Now be very honest and ask yourself, "How sure am I that I can really do this?" Use the following scale to represent your degree of certainty:

1	2	3	4	5	6	7	8	9	10
Very unlikely				Possibly		Probably			Definitely

If your answer is at the upper end of the scale, your goal is too easy. This might be the case if you and your friend live next door to each other. However, suppose she or he lives three miles away and you have arthritis in your hip. Your degree of certainty will be very low on the scale. Aim for a goal that gives you a "certainty reading" of 7–8. Your contract partner can also make a similar commitment about something he or she wants to do. This is a very powerful method of changing behavior and achieving goals in all areas of your life. Give it a try!

Points to Remember

- Make a commitment to exercise.
- Be realistic about your goals.
- Start with small, easily achievable amounts of exercise and build up gradually and steadily.
- Include a variety of activities.
- Exercise with other people sometimes.
- Do not do any exercise that causes severe pain or discomfort.
- You have done too much if you experience exercise-induced pain for more than about two hours.
- Do not exercise a painful, inflamed joint.
- Consult a physical therapist or doctor if you are doubtful about an exercise.
- Congratulate yourself on taking such a positive step in *learning to live* with your arthritis.

4

Morning Wake-Up

Do you find that your joints are stiff and difficult to move when you wake up in the morning? This is a common problem, particularly for people with rheumatoid arthritis.

Morning Wake-Up is a sequence of exercises that move all the main joints of your body. This will help to get you moving and out of bed in the morning.

How you feel when you wake up often depends on how well you slept and rested during the night. A good night's sleep is really important. It's much harder to cope with aches and pains if you are tired.

You should give your body the best support possible with a good firm mattress. A low pillow is preferable, especially if you have neck problems. A light down-filled comforter provides as much warmth as three or four blankets and eases the weight on your body through the night. It also makes it a lot easier to make the bed!

A bed that has been nicely warmed up by an electric blanket is comforting to climb into.

Getting to sleep or waking up during the night can be a worry. There are no easy solutions, but we have included a few suggestions in "Relaxation" (page 119). Give them a try.

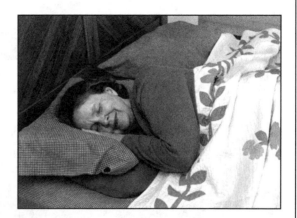

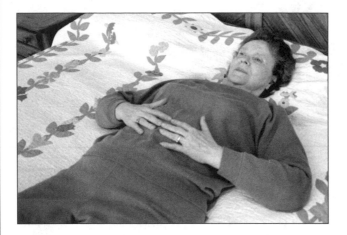

1. Start: Lie with hands on your lower ribs.

1a. Breathe in slowly and easily. Feel your chest expand under your hands. Let your breath out in a sigh.

1b. Open your mouth wide and yawn.

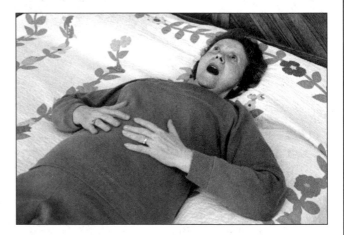

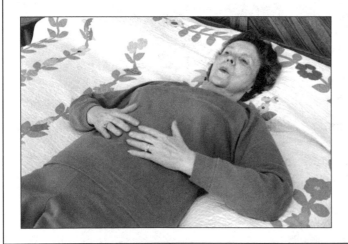

1c. Breathe in, then gently blow the air out. Continue blowing out until your lungs are empty; let yourself breathe in.

However, even after a really good night's sleep, you may still wake up feeling that you can't move. This is when you need Morning Wake-Up to help get yourself up and about.

Make sure you give yourself about 10–15 minutes to go slowly through the whole sequence. You must gently encourage your joints to move, not force them. Do each of the movements two or three times, maybe an extra couple of times for your stiffest joints. You can include exercises from other parts of the book if you think they would be particularly helpful. If you are running short of time in the morning, just do the breathing (Exercise 1), and then choose the exercises that move your problem joints.

Getting out of bed is easier when you use the method shown in Exercise 10. In this way, you use the body's own momentum, which puts less strain on your joints.

In some of the pictures we have left the sheets and blankets off the model so you can see what she is doing. However, it is important for you to keep warm, so don't follow her example. Keep under the covers. Just make sure they are loose enough so that you can move easily.

Have a good morning!

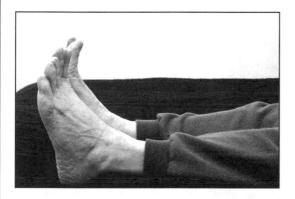

2. Start: Lie with your legs straight.
2a. Bend back your toes.

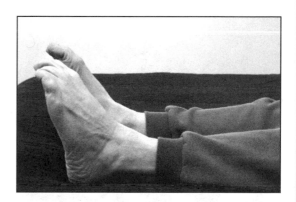

2b. Gently curl your toes under.

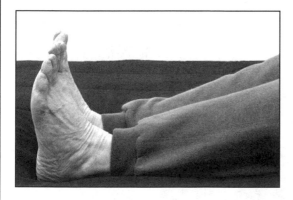

2c. Bend back your foot.

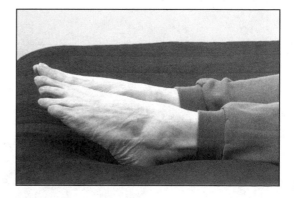

2d. Push your foot down.

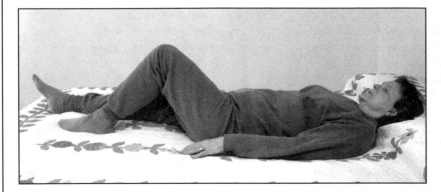

3. Start: Lie with your legs straight.

Slide your heel up toward your bottom. Straighten your leg out along the bed. Repeat with the other leg.

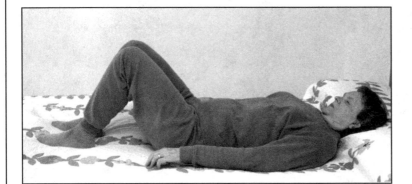

4. Start: Lie with both knees bent.

4a. Gently arch your back.

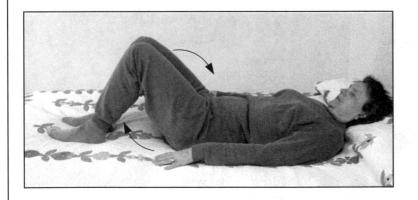

4b. Flatten your back onto the bed and tilt your pelvis upward by tightening your buttocks and stomach muscles.

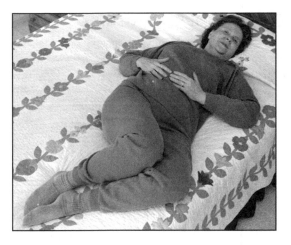

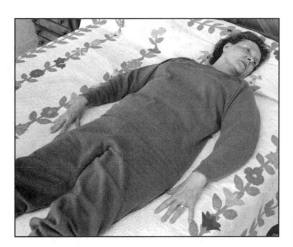

5. Start: Lie with both knees bent.
Gently roll your knees from side to side.

6. Start: Lie looking upward.
Gently roll your head from side to side.

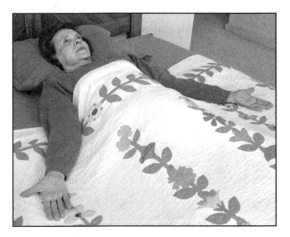

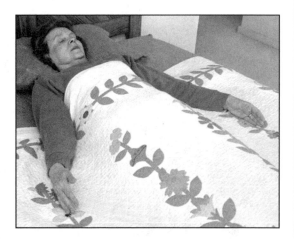

7. Start: Lie with your arms by your sides.
7a. Gently roll your arms outward, turning your palms up.

7b. Gently roll your arms inward, turning your palms down and then outward.

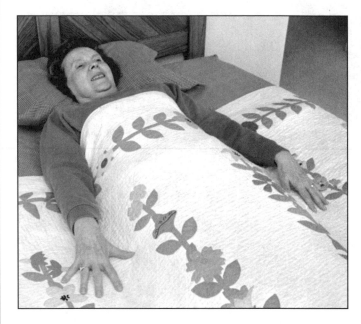

8. Start: Lie with your arms by your sides.
8a. Stretch out your fingers.

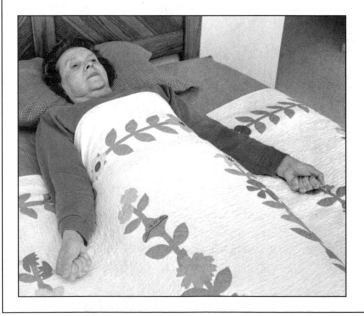

8b. Gently curl your fingers into your palm.

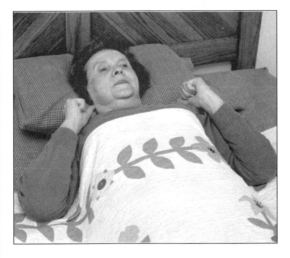

9. Start: Lie with your hands by your sides on top of the blankets.

9a. Gently curl up your fingers and bring your fists to your shoulders.

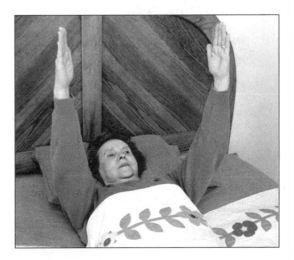

9b. Stretch your arms upward, opening out your fingers.

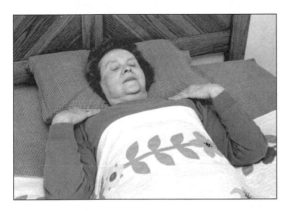

9c. Lower your elbows to the bed and touch your shoulders with your fingertips.

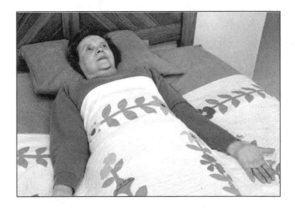

9d. Straighten your arms down by your sides.

Getting Out of Bed

10. Start: Lie with both knees bent up. Use a continuous flowing movement.

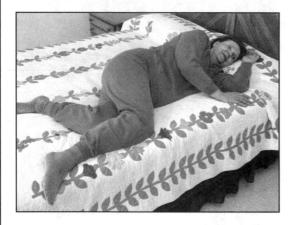

10a. Roll to one side, stretching across your body with the top arm.

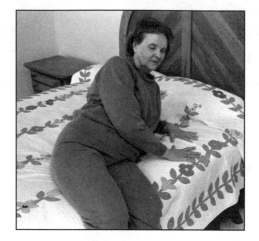

10b–d. Pivot on your bottom so your legs swing down over the edge of the bed and your body swings upward. Assist the movement, pushing with your top hand and bottom elbow.

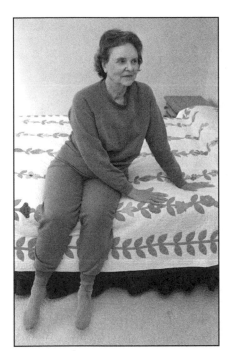 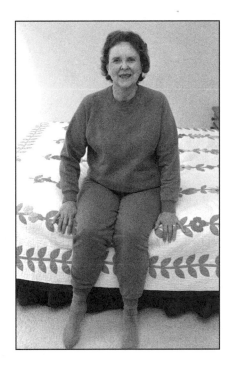

5

Warm–Up

It is a good idea to warm up your whole body before you start doing exercises for your specific problem areas—particularly if you have been sitting still for a while. Arthritic joints can stiffen up very easily. Warming up may also include some of the pre-exercise techniques discussed on page 20.

This Warm-Up sequence is a gentle way of starting to move. It helps to get both you and your joints into the mood for exercise. Once your muscles start working, your circulation increases. It is the blood that transports oxygen, energy, and nourishment to your body and takes away the waste products. As the circulation to your joints and

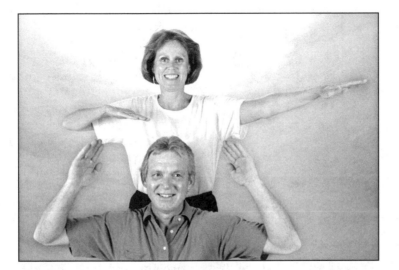

43

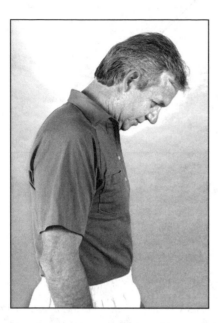

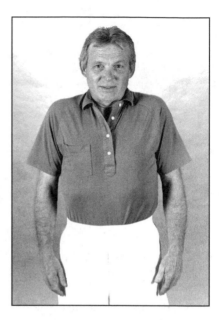

Start your Warm-Up with five slow full breaths. Let each breath out completely.

1. Start: Breathe in.

Breathe <u>out</u> as you bend your head forward. Breathe <u>in</u> as you lift your head up. <u>Do not bend your head backward.</u>

2. Start: Look straight ahead.

Breathe <u>in</u> as you lift up your shoulders.

Breathe <u>out</u> as you relax your shoulders.

muscles increases, they warm up and are able to move more easily. This means you can gradually work up to more difficult exercises after starting with some easy movements.

As we have said, your whole body needs exercise, not just those joints that are giving you trouble. Remember, regular exercise will help prevent further problems. If you are very short of time one day, just doing the Warm-Up will ensure that you have moved all the main joints of your body.

You can do the Warm-Up either sitting on a chair or standing up. It depends on which you find most comfortable.

Exercises 1–6 can all be done sitting or standing. If you want to remain sitting, finish with Exercises 7 and 8. If you don't mind weight bearing, then add Exercises 9 and 10.

Do each exercise 2–4 times.

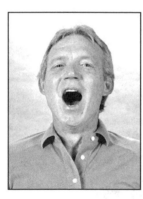

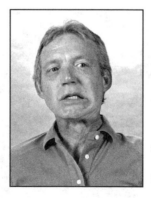

3. Start with your mouth closed.

3a. Stretch your mouth open and let yourself yawn.

3b. Imagine you are chewing a large piece of sticky toffee. Stretch your mouth in all directions for 5–10 seconds.

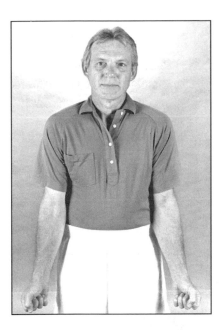

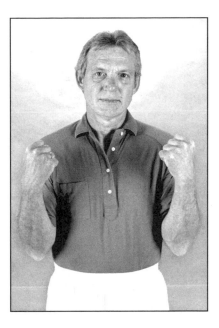

4. Start: Sit or stand with your arms by your sides.
4a. Curl your fingers into a loose fist.

4b. Bring your hands up to your shoulders.

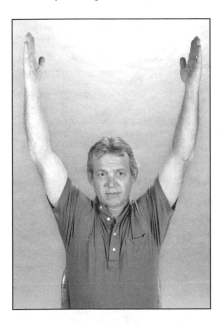

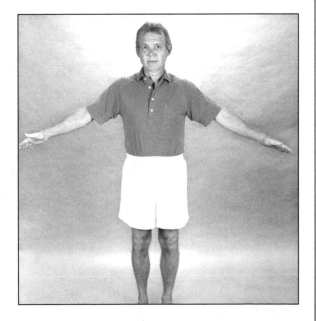

4c. Spread open your fingers as you stretch your arms upward, with your palms facing each other.

4d. Lower your arms sideways, with your palms facing downward.

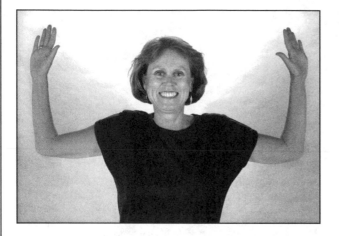

5. Start: Sit or stand with your arms held out to the sides, elbows at right angles, and palms facing forward. Keep your elbows at shoulder level.

15a. Breathe <u>in</u> as you stretch backward with your arms.

5b. Breathe <u>out</u> as you bring your elbows and palms together.

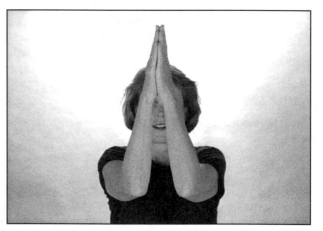

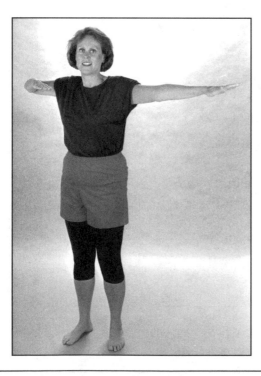

6. Start: Sit or stand, looking straight ahead.

Stretch forward with one arm and backward with the other elbow. Let yourself twist at the waist. Look at your front hand. Change arms and twist the other way.

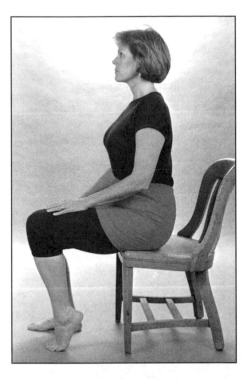

7. Start: Sit with both feet flat on the floor.
Lift the heel of each foot alternately.

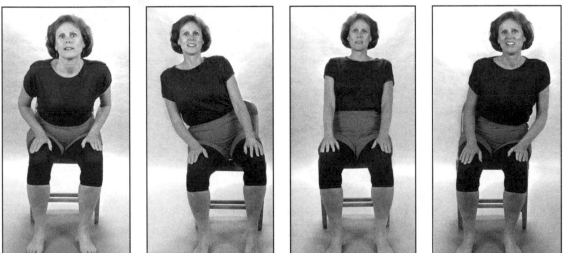

8. Start: Sit up straight with both feet flat on the floor.
Keep your feet on the floor and your back straight. Rock your body around in a circle.

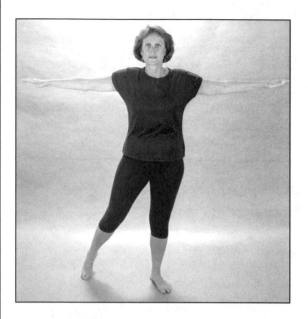

9. Start: Stand with feet apart.

9a. Breathe <u>in</u> as you rock your weight over onto one leg and lift your arms out sideways.

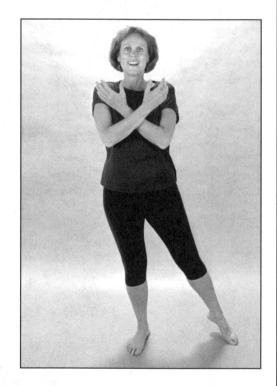

9b. Breathe <u>out</u> as you rock over onto the other leg and swing your arms down and across your body.

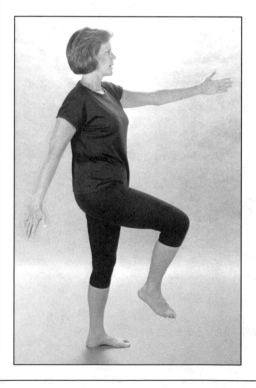

10. Start: Stand with your feet together and arms by your sides.

Mark time by stretching one arm forward and the other arm backward. Lift the opposite knee to the forward arm. Change arms and legs.

6

Neck

You might well call someone who keeps bothering you a "pain in the neck." This common usage suggests just how troublesome neck pain can be.

The neck is the upper part of the spine and is made up of seven bones, or vertebrae, stacked one on top of each other. They all work together to allow your head to move in many directions.

Pain in the neck can be caused by various things—one of which is arthritis. Actual arthritis in the neck means that the joints between the vertebrae have been affected.

Arthritis in the neck is often associated with one-sided headaches or pain, numbness, and tingling down one arm. This is called "referred pain." It is due to irritation of the nerves going up to your head or down your arm.

The neck has a large range of movement. This means that we can easily watch what is going on around us. You have probably found that life is more difficult with a stiff neck. However, greater mobility means a sacrifice in stability. So the muscles and

ligaments that support the neck are easily strained and overstretched. For instance, this is what happens when you twist your neck or sleep in an unusual position. Also, in a whiplash injury the head is swung

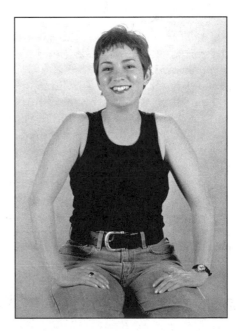

uncontrollably forward and backward. The joints are forced way beyond their normal limits, damaging the supporting soft tissues of the neck.

We often carry a lot of general tension in the muscles around the neck and upper back, making a neck problem worse. If the muscles are tense or in spasm, they tend to squash the joints of the neck together, causing more pain. Of course, pain in the neck can also lead to increased tension in the muscles, thus creating a cycle of pain and tension. Tension in the muscles of the head and neck often result in a headache.

Your head is quite heavy. It weighs about 10 lbs (4 1/2 kg)! A lot of effort is needed to hold it upright. You will put less strain on your neck if you keep it lengthened and in line with the rest of your body (see "Posture," p. 126).

Avoid any movement that tends to squash the vertebrae together. This means any exercise that makes your head bend backward. Also, be aware of how you hold your head. Do you have your chin poking forward? This position puts the same stress on the joints of your neck as bending your head backward. Imagine that the *crown* of your head is attached to a balloon, and let your head float like the balloon. But don't try too hard to hold your head in the correct position. This will only increase the strain. Exercise 2 will help to improve the way you balance your head on your neck.

You may wonder why we have included eye exercises in the neck section. The reason is that you can take some of the strain off a sore and stiff neck by making your eyes do some of the work for you.

A final word of caution: the neck is a delicate part of the body, so be careful with these exercises. If any of them causes markedly increased neck pain or pain, numbness, or tingling radiating down your arm, then don't do them.

Start with 2–4 repetitions of each exercise.

The key exercises for this section are 2, 3, 4, 5, and 6.

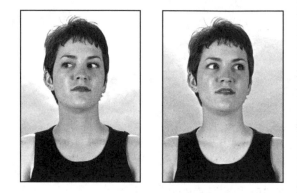

1. Start: Look straight ahead. Keep your head still throughout.

1a, b. Move only your eyes and look from side to side.

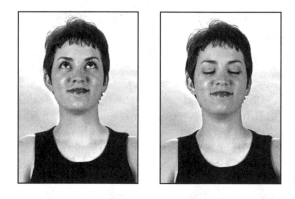

1c, d. Move only your eyes and look up and down.

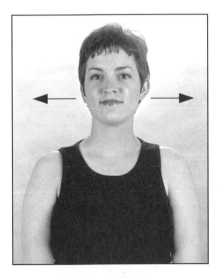

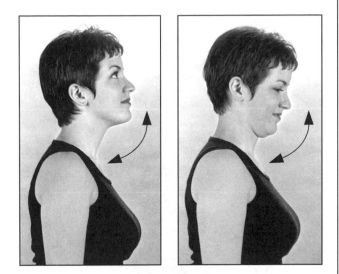

*2a. Start: Imagine you have a horizontal line (axis) going through your head, just behind your earlobes.

2b, c. Nod your head up and down around this axis without moving your neck. Finish with your chin slightly dropped.

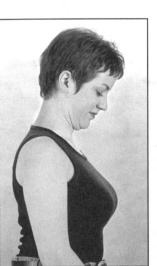

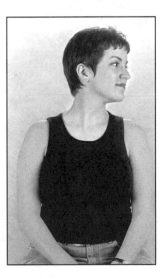

* 3. Start: Look straight ahead with your chin slightly dropped.

Bend your head forward, keeping your chin tucked in. Straighten up but <u>do not bend your head backwards.</u>

*4. Start: Look straight ahead, with your chin slightly dropped.

Turn your head and look over alternate shoulders.

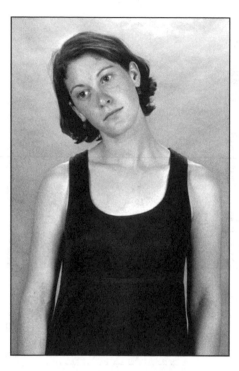

*5. Start: Look straight ahead with your chin slightly dropped.
Keep looking straight ahead and bend your head sideways, taking your ear toward your shoulder. <u>Do not</u> lift your shoulder. Bend your head to the other side.

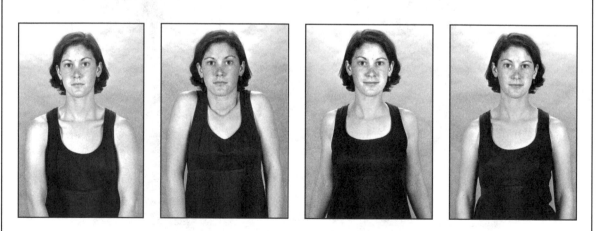

*6. Start: Look straight ahead with your shoulders relaxed.
6a-d. Roll your shoulders in a circular movement—forward, up, backward, and down.

Arms

Here are some exercises for your shoulders and elbows. These joints are more commonly affected by rheumatoid arthritis than by osteoarthritis. They are also common sites for bursitis and tendonitis.

The shoulder is the most flexible joint in your body. Normally it is able to perform many complex movements. If there is any injury to a shoulder joint, it may try to protect itself from further hurt by becoming "frozen."

A frozen shoulder can become permanently stiff if it is not exercised properly. Concentrate on Exercises 1–2 if the amount of movement in your shoulder is very limited. These are gentle exercises that will gradually help to increase your shoulder mobility. If your shoulders are reasonably mobile, don't bother with these. Start with Exercise 3.

It doesn't matter whether you sit or stand to do these arm exercises—do whichever you find more comfortable.

Start with 2–4 repetitions of each exercise.

The key arm exercises are 4, 5, and 6.

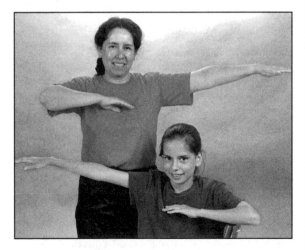

1. Start: Lean forward with one hand on a table or the back of a chair. Let the opposite arm hang down. Let the weight of your arm do the swinging like a pendulum; do not let the movement get out of control.

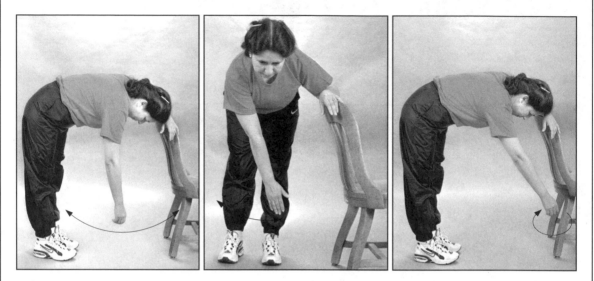

1a. Swing your arm gently forward and back, like a pendulum.

1b. Swing your arm gently out and across your body, like a pendulum.

1c. Swing your arm around in small circles. Reverse direction.

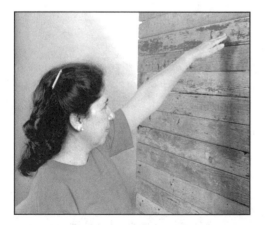

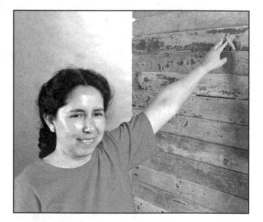

2. Start: Stand about half an arm's length away from a wall.

2a. Face the wall. Walk your fingers upward as far as you can.

2b. Stand with your side to the wall. Walk your fingers up as far as you can.

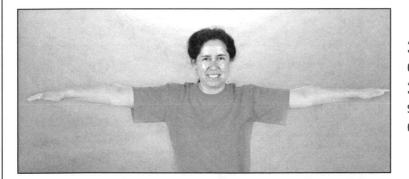

3. Start: Sit or stand with your arms by your sides.

3a. Lift both arms out sideways to shoulder level, palms facing downward.

3b. Keep your arms at shoulder level. Bend one elbow and touch the front of your shoulder.

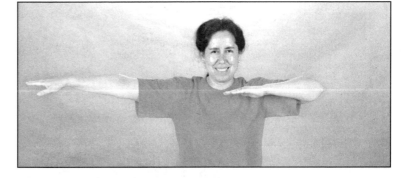

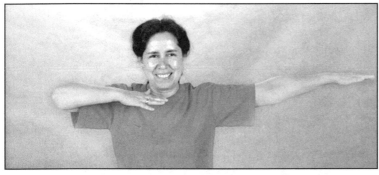

3c. Straighten this arm and bend the other elbow.

3d. Straighten out both arms, and then lower them slowly to your sides.

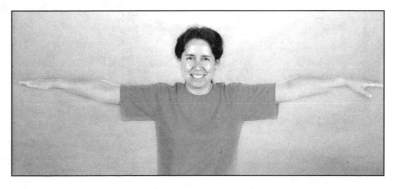

*4. Start: Sit or stand with your arms by your sides, palms facing backward.

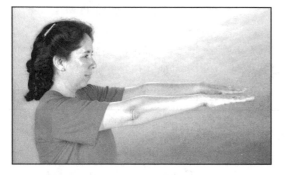

4a. Lift both arms forward to shoulder level, palms facing down.

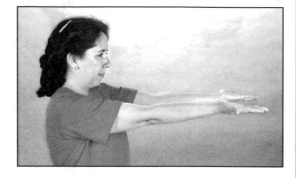

4b. Turn your palms up.

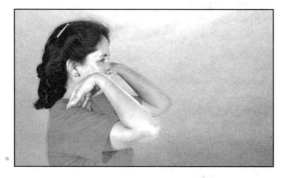

4c. Touch your fingertips to your shoulders, letting your elbows drop.

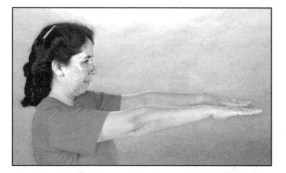

4d. Stretch both arms forward at shoulder level, turning your palms down.

4e. Lower your arms slowly and stretch behind your back. Try to touch your palms together.

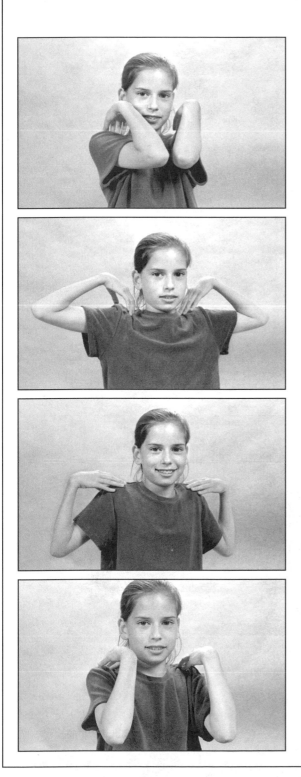

*5. Start with your fingertips touching your shoulders.

5a–d. Make large circles with your elbows, bringing them forward, up, back, and down. <u>Breathe in</u> as you open up and back; <u>breathe out</u> as you close down and forward.

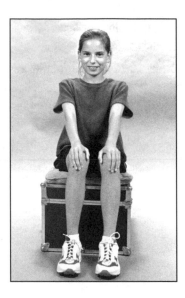

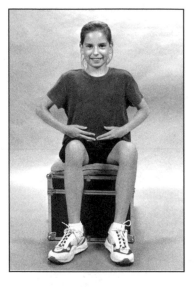

*6. Start: Sit with your back straight and your feet flat.

6a. Stretch your hands down to touch your knees.

6b. Touch your stomach, keeping your elbows out to the side.

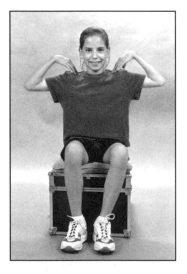

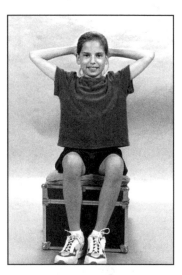

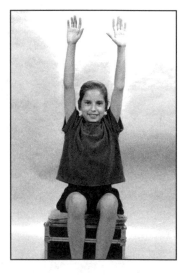

6c. Touch your shoulders, with your elbows lifted out to the side.

6d. Touch behind your head.

6e. Stretch both arms upward, palms facing each other. Lower your arms with the reverse movements.

Hands

We use our hands for so many activities that any pain or limitation of movement is soon noticed. Hands are made up of two basic parts with somewhat different functions: the wrist and the fingers.

The main purpose of the wrist is to provide a stable platform from which the much more delicate and mobile fingers can operate. The strength of your hands and fingers is influenced by the position of your wrist. Notice how your wrist bends backward as you make a fist. A stiff wrist can affect the function of your whole hand.

The large number of finger joints give the fingers their mobility and manipulative ability. They can also compensate for each other to some extent. This means that your hands can still be quite functional even though you have a few stiff joints.

Osteoarthritis usually affects the end joints of the fingers, and you may develop knobby swellings over these joints. They may not look very good, but usually they are not very troublesome.

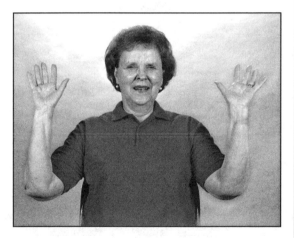

Rheumatoid arthritis in the hands, however, may cause more severe problems. But don't panic—these don't necessarily occur! The joints of the hands most commonly affected by rheumatoid arthritis are the wrists, the knuckles, and the middle joints of the fingers. Sometimes the disease process can cause so much damage to the delicate tendons and ligaments that they no longer support the joint in the correct position. Hand deformities can then develop. The most common of these, called *ulnar deviation,* occurs when the hands and fingers start to bend, or deviate, away from the thumb. If this is happening to your hands, be sure to concentrate on Exercise 8.

If you are having lots of problems with your fingers, exercise each hand separately.

Use your other hand to gently assist the movement. But *be careful* not to force your fingers. Your hands are very delicate and need to be coaxed gently into action.

Start with 2–4 repetitions of each exercise.

The key exercises are 1, 4, and 6.

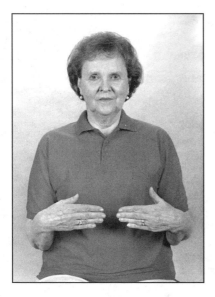

*1. Start with your elbows tucked in and your palms facing each other.

1a. Bend your wrists forward, bringing your fingers toward each other.

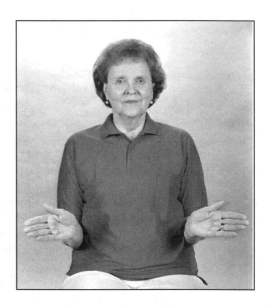

1b. Bend your wrists back so that your palms face the front.

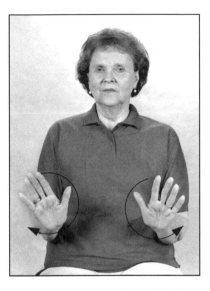
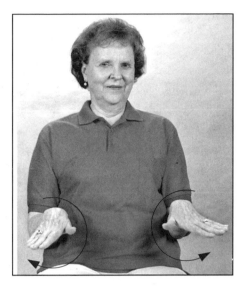

2. Start with your elbows tucked in.

2a–c. Circle your hands inward from the wrist—up, in, down, and out.

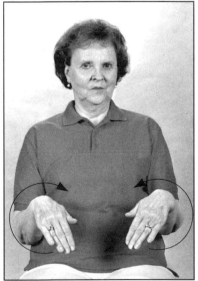

3. Between exercises: relax your fingers by playing an imaginary piano with your fingers and thumb.

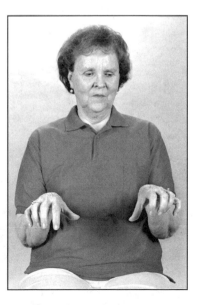

*4. Start with your hands in front of you, looking at your palms.

4a. Stretch your thumb across your palm and <u>gently</u> close your fingers over it.

4b. Stretch open your fingers and thumb.

4c. <u>Gently</u> fold your fingers into your palm and close your thumb over them. <u>Do not make a tight fist.</u>

Stretch open your fingers and thumb again.

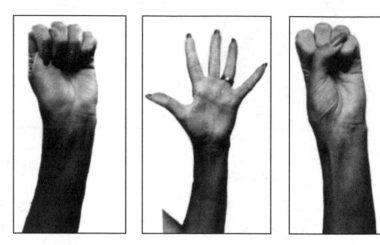

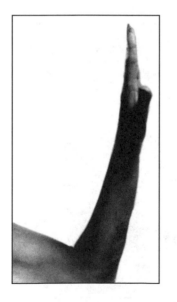

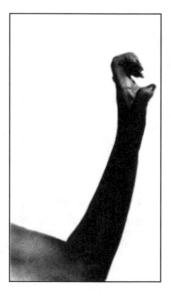

5. Start with your hands in front of you, palms facing each other.

5a. Straighten out your fingers and thumb.

5b. Bend the top two joints of your fingers down towards the top of your palms. Keep the knuckle joint straight. If your fingers are very stiff, bend each finger individually, helping with the other hand.

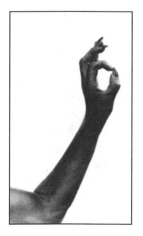 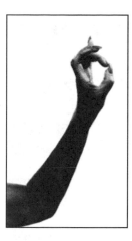 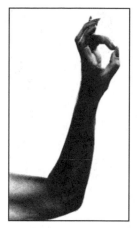 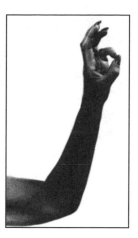

*6. Start: Do each hand individually.

6a–d. Touch the tip of your thumb to the tip of each finger in turn. Make the circle as round as you can. Straighten your fingers in between touching each finger.

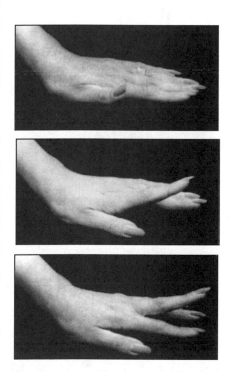

7. Start: Place your hands on a table with your palms down.

7a. Lift your thumb up off the table, then replace it.

7b–e. Lift each finger up off the table, one at a time.

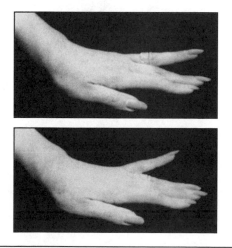

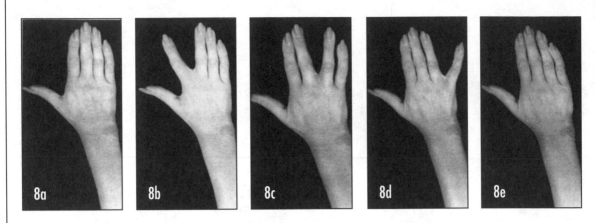

8. Start: Place your hands on a table with your palms down.

8a. Stretch your thumb away from your fingers.

8b–e. Move each finger individually toward your thumb.

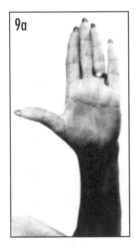
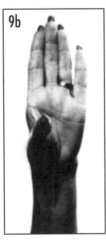
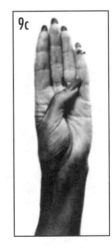

9 Start: Look at the palms of your hands.

9a. Stretch your thumb out sideways away from your palm.

9b. Stretch your thumb forward away from your palm.

9c. Stretch your thumb across your palm to touch the base of your little finger.

Back

Your back is the central support for your whole body and as such must be both strong and flexible. This dual function is achieved by the column of 24 separate bones (called vertebrae) stacked one on top of the other. Each vertebra is separated from its neighbor, above and below, by a spongy shock-absorbing disc. There are also lots of strong ligaments and muscles supporting your spine.

Straining your back means that you have probably damaged a ligament or muscle. Usually this does not pose much of a long-term problem. A more serious back complaint is what is commonly called a *slipped disc.* This is not a very accurate term since the disc has not actually slipped out of place. Rather, what has happened is that some of the jelly-like substance inside the disc has been squeezed out. This can irritate one of the nerves going down to your leg.

If you have pain radiating down the back of your leg or any numbness, tingling, or muscle weakness in your leg, you have probably been told you have *sciatica.* All

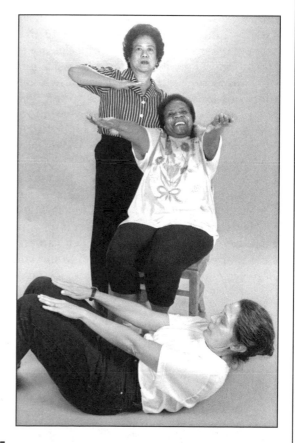

this means is that the sciatic nerve, which runs down from your lower back, across your buttock, and down the back of your leg, is being irritated. It may be because of a slipped disc, but in older people it's usually due to arthritis in the joints of the lower back. As we get older the discs become a bit squashed, so the spaces between the vertebrae are narrower. Osteoarthritis in the lower back may result in small bony spurs growing on the edges of the vertebrae. Both these conditions can cause irritation to the nerves.

When your back is in an acute stage of injury or inflammation, the muscles of the back may go into spasm. This is your back's way of protecting you from further pain or injury. However, the muscle spasm itself can be quite painful, resulting in further muscle tension. If your back muscles are in spasm, then you should rest your back and only do very gentle exercises. Remember that your muscles are trying to protect you.

If your back problem is more chronic or if you want to prevent another injury, regular exercise to build up the muscles supporting your back is essential. You have to take good care of your back, too! This means maintaining good posture (refer to page 126) and lifting correctly (refer to page 129).

Two main sets of muscle support your back: *your back muscles,* which you can feel on either side of your spine and, would you believe, *your stomach muscles!* Stomach muscles are particularly important in maintaining good posture and in preventing swayback. For chronic low back pain, probably the best exercise is the pelvic tilt (Exercises 6–8). This exercise can be done in various positions. Try all the variations or choose the one you find most comfortable.

If you have osteoporosis of the spine, take care with exercises that bend you forward or sideways (Exercises 2, 3, 5).

We have included some back exercises to be done on hands and knees (Exercises 16–21). Do not do these exercises if you have problems with your shoulders, wrists, or knees—all the movements are covered in other exercises.

We have also included a section of exercises specifically for people with ankylosing spondylitis (Exercises 18–21). These include a number designed to arch your spine backward, since ankylosing spondylitis tends to bend you forward. Anyone can do these exercises, but *be very careful.* Stop doing them if you experience increased back pain.

Start with 2–4 repetitions of each exercise. Cut down or eliminate any exercise that you feel increases your back pain or causes pain going down your leg. After a while you will be able to decide which of these exercises are most beneficial for your particular back problem.

The key exercises in this section are 1, 3, 4, 6, 7, 8, and 11.

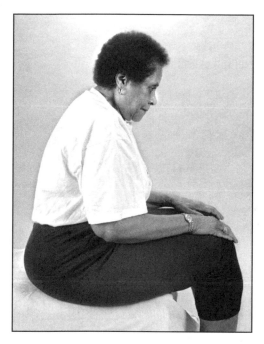

* 1. Start: Sit with your feet flat.

Caution: Do this exercise very carefully if you have a hip replacement.

Keep your back and neck in a straight line. Rock forward and then upright as though you are hinged at the hips.

2. Start: Sit with your feet flat.

Caution: Do not do this exercise if you have a hip replacement. Take care if you have osteoporosis of the spine or neck.

Bend your head forward, then slowly curl your body forward, taking your forehead toward your knees. Slowly uncurl from the bottom of your spine until you are sitting upright. Relax your shoulders.

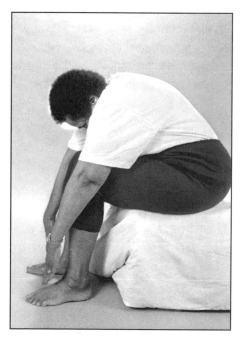

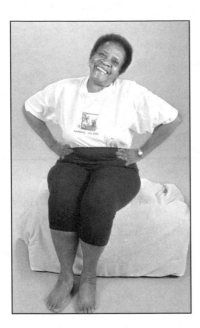

*3. Start: Sit with your feet flat and your hands on your waist.

Caution: Take care if you have osteoporosis of the spine.

Keep looking straight ahead and bend your trunk to one side, over your hand. Straighten up and bend to the other side.

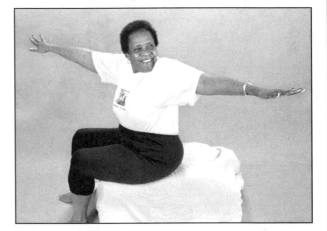

* 4. Start: Sit with your feet flat and your arms held out to the side.

4a. Turn your head to look at one hand. Keep looking at your hand as you take your arm backward, twisting from the waist. Return to face forward, and then twist to the other side.

4b. Keep looking straight ahead as you take one arm backward, twisting from the waist. Return to the front, and then take your other arm back.

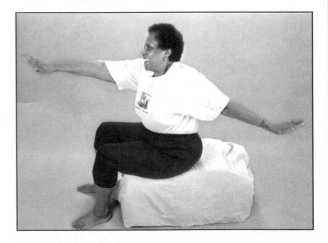

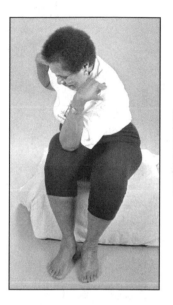

5. Start: Sit with your feet apart and your fingertips on your shoulders.

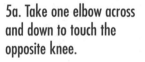

Caution: Do not do this exercise if you have a hip replacement. Take care if you have osteoporosis of the spine.

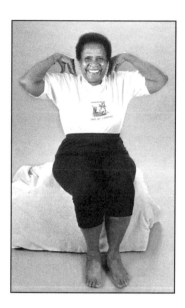

5a. Take one elbow across and down to touch the opposite knee.

5b. Straighten up and gently stretch both elbows backward. Repeat to the other side.

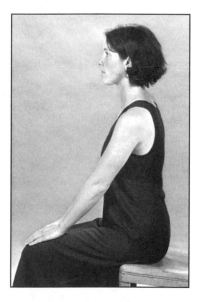

Pelvic rock: The movement is one of 'rocking' your pelvis backward and forward. Do not move your upper body.

*6. Start: Sit up straight with your feet on the floor.

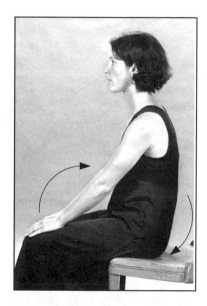

6a. Gently arch your lower back. (Rock your pelvis backward.)

6b. Tuck your pelvis under by tightening your buttocks and stomach muscles. (Rock your pelvis forward.)

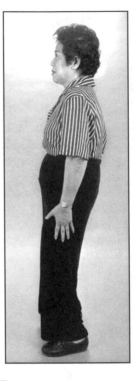
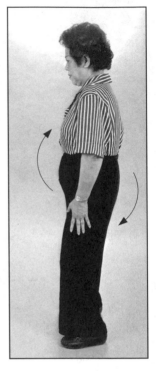

*7. Start: Stand with your feet hip-width apart, knees loose, hands on your hips.

7a. Gently arch your lower back. (Rock backward.)

7b. Tuck your pelvis under by tightening your buttocks and stomach muscles. (Rock forward.)

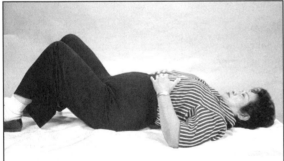

*8. Start: Lie on your back on the floor with both knees bent.

8a. Gently arch your lower back off the floor. (Rock backward.)

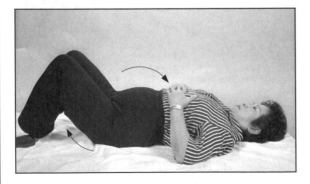

8b. Tuck your pelvis under and flatten your lower back by tightening your buttocks and stomach muscles. (Rock forward.)

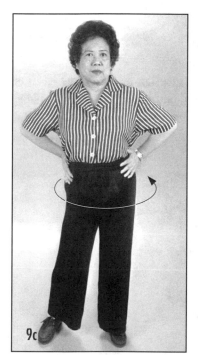

9a

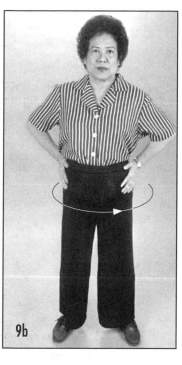

9b

9. Start: Stand with your feet hip-width apart, hands on your hips. Keep your knees loose.

> **Caution:** Do this exercise very carefully if you have sciatica or a severe back condition.

9a–d. Roll your pelvis around in a circle, taking it sideways, forward, to the other side, and backward. Move from your waist and keep your upper body still. Roll your pelvis around in the other direction.

9c

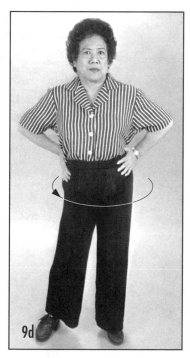

9d

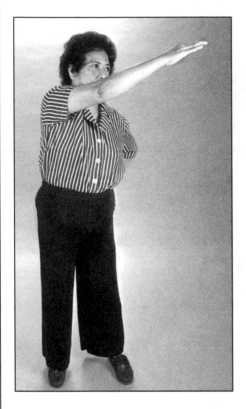

10. Start: Stand with your feet apart and hands on your waist.

Keeping both feet flat, stretch one arm up and across your body. Let your body twist and look at your hand. Repeat to the other side.

*11. Start: Lie on your back with your knees bent and hands on your thighs.

Caution: If you have problems with your neck, use a pillow.

Tuck your chin in. Lift your shoulders by sliding your hands up toward your knees. Lower slowly, keeping your chin tucked in.

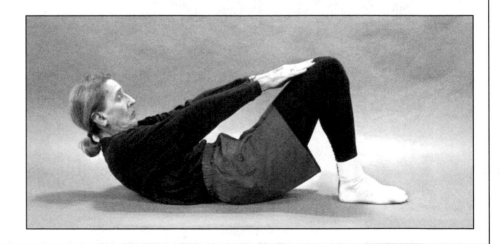

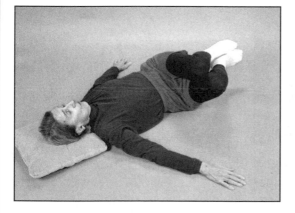

12. Start: Lie on your back with your knees bent and your feet apart.

> **Caution:** If you have problems with your neck, use a pillow.

Tuck your chin in and lift your shoulders to one side by sliding both hands up toward one knee. Lower slowly, keeping your chin tucked in. Repeat to the other side.

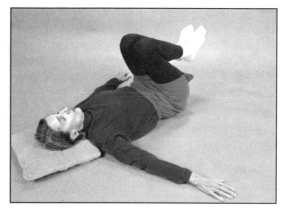

13a. Start: Lie on your back with both knees bent up toward your chest. Stretch both arms out sideways.

> **Caution:** Do not do this exercise if you have a hip replacement.

13b. Take both knees over to one side. Do not go farther than half-way to the floor. Repeat to the other side.

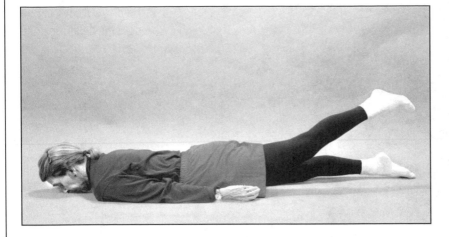

14. Start: Lie on your front with your hands by your sides.

Lift one leg up off the floor, with the knee straight. Keep both front hip bones on the floor.

15. Start: Lie on your back with your knees bent up toward your chest and your hands on your knees.

Caution: Take care with this exercise if you have a hip replacement.

15a–d. Massage your lower back by gently rocking around in small circles. Circle in both directions.

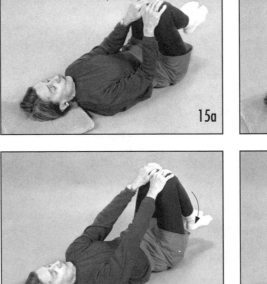

15a

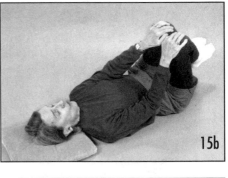

15b

15c

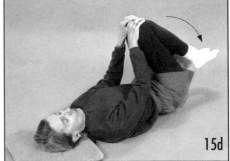

15d

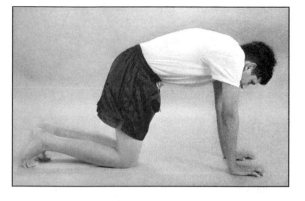

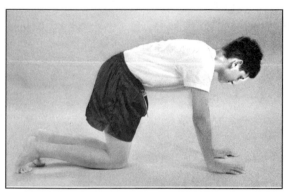

16. Start on hands and knees with your hands under your shoulders and your knees under your hips.

16a. Tuck under your head and your tail, and arch upward with your back.

16b. Lower slowly and flatten your back. Do not let your back arch downward.

17. Start on hands and knees.

Without moving your head, "wag your tail" from side to side. Do not arch your back.

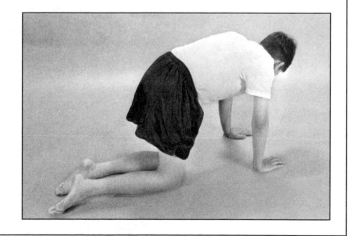

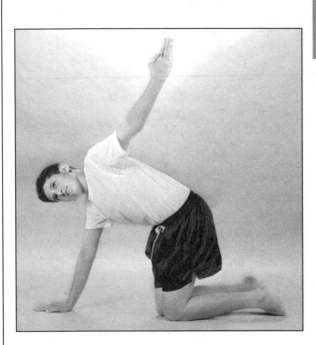

18. Start on your hands and knees with your hands under your shoulders and knees under your hips.

Look at one hand as you lift it out to the side and upward, letting your spine twist.

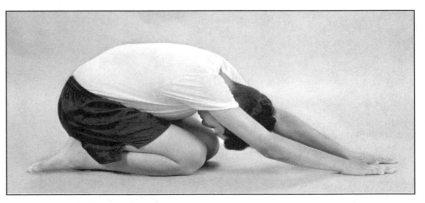

19. Start on your hands and knees.

Without moving your hands, stretch your bottom back toward your heels. Hold the stretch for about five seconds.

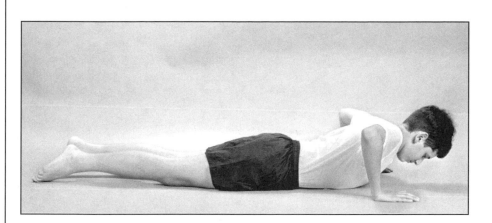

20. Start: Lie on your front with your hands under your shoulders.

Lift up your head and then push up through your hands to lift your shoulders only. Keep your chest on the floor. Hold for a few seconds before lowering slowly.

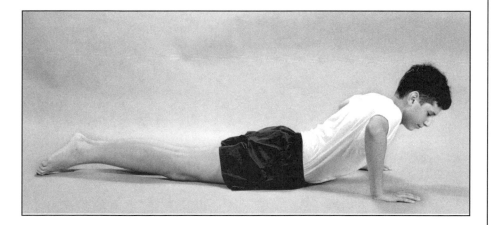

21. Start: Lie on your front with your hands under your shoulders.

Lift up your head and then push up through your hands and lift up your chest. Keep your front hipbones on the floor. Hold for a few seconds before lowering slowly.

Hips

The hip joint is a ball and socket joint—made up of a ball part on the end of the thigh bone that fits into a curved socket in the pelvis. It is a joint that needs a large range of movement, combined with the strength and stability required to bear the weight of your body. The joint is well supported by those large strong muscles of your upper and outer thighs and your buttocks.

The hip is a common site for arthritis, both osteoarthritis and rheumatoid arthritis. You may feel the pain from an arthritic hip in the groin or the upper or outer thigh, or even referred down to the knee or below. If you have arthritis in your hip, you need to build up the strength of the muscles supporting it. You have to keep mobile too, so that you can put on your socks and tie up your shoelaces.

Nowadays, complete hip replacements are quite common and usually very successful. This may be a solution if your hip pain is chronic and severe. If you have had

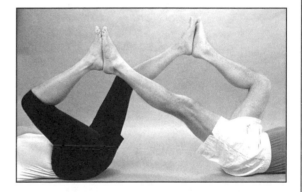

a hip replacement, it's very important that you strengthen the muscles that provide support for your hip. There are, however, some movements that you must avoid because they endanger the stability of your artificial hip. You should not bend your hip more than 90°, and you should not cross the leg with the hip replacement over in front of your other leg. One of the worst things you can do is to sit with your legs crossed!

If you have a hip replacement, take note of the cautions on Exercises 1 and 4.

If you have difficulty getting down onto the floor, just do the sitting and standing exercises.

Start by doing 2–4 repetitions of each exercise.

The key hip exercises are 3, 4, and 7.

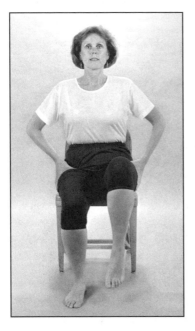

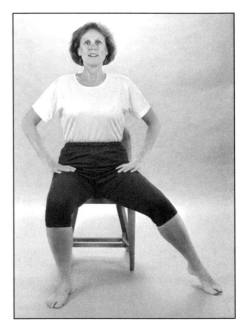

1. Start: Sit on a chair with both feet on the floor.

> **Caution:** Be careful if you have a hip replacement.

Keep your back straight and lift up one knee. Lower slowly, and then repeat with the other leg.

2. Start: Sit with your feet flat.

Keep your body still and lift one leg out to the side, then back in. Repeat with the other leg.

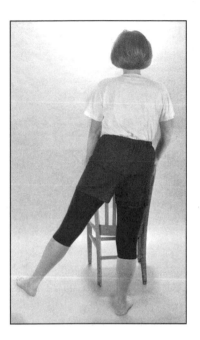

*3. Start: Stand, holding onto the back of a chair with both hands.

Keep your body upright as you lift one leg out to the side, with your foot flexed and toes pointing forward. Lower slowly and repeat with the other leg.

*4. Start: Stand, holding onto the back of a chair with one hand.

Caution: Do not lift your leg above hip level if you have a hip replacement.

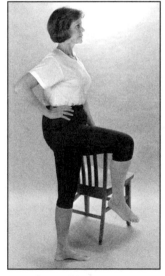

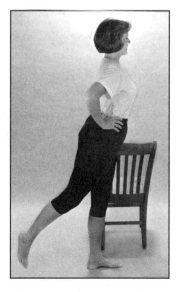

4a. Keep your back straight and lift up your outside knee.

4b. Straighten your knee as you stretch your leg behind you, with your toes just off the floor. Turn around to work the other leg.

5. Start: Lie on your back with your legs out straight.

Keep your leg straight and your toes pointing upward. Slide one leg out to the side and then back in. Repeat with the other leg.

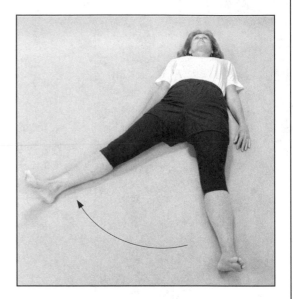

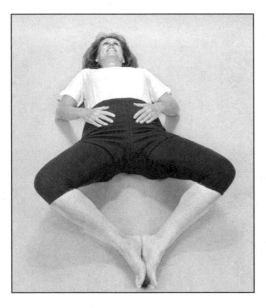

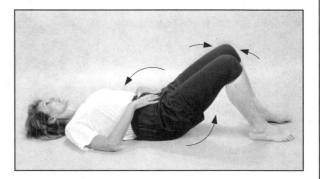

6. Start: Lie on your back with your knees bent and your feet together.

6a. Keep your feet together and slowly stretch your knees apart.

6b. Close your knees and press them together as you tilt your pelvis upward (refer to back exercises 6–8)— tighten your buttocks and your stomach muscles.

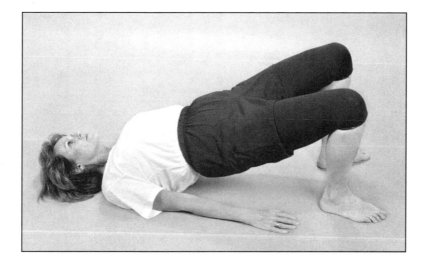

*7. Start: Lie on your back with your knees bent and your feet and knees comfortably apart.

Push through your feet and slowly lift your bottom off the floor. Lower slowly, rolling your spine onto the floor from the top downward.

Knees

The knee is a common problem site for people with arthritis, both osteoarthritis and rheumatoid arthritis. The knee joint acts like a hinge—it can only bend and straighten. It needs to be strong since it is being used constantly during normal daily activities. The knee acts as one of the main shock absorbers for the jarring that occurs each time we take a step.

The large muscle in the front of your thigh is known as the quadriceps muscle. It is this muscle that straightens and supports your knee and holds you upright. Therefore it is crucial that this muscle is strong. If your knees feel weak or give way, then concentrate on Exercises 1, 2, and 7, which will strengthen the quadriceps muscle.

Arthritic knees can sometimes look a bit unsightly. They may become large and puffy-looking, or you may be knock-kneed or bowlegged. This does not mean that they have to be less functional, though. Some people are unable to straighten their knees completely, or they may have unstable, wobbly joints.

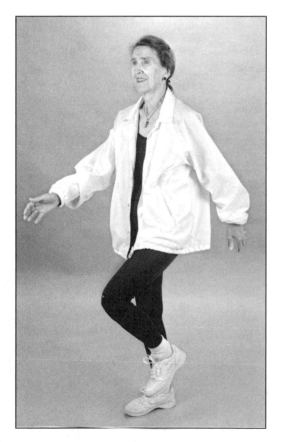

If your knees have any of these problems, concentrate on strengthening the quadriceps muscles to give your knees as much support as possible (Exercises 1, 2, and 7).

If you have particularly painful or unstable knees, omit Exercises 4, 5, and 6: they may put too much strain on your knees.

Knee replacements are becoming more common these days. If you have a knee replacement, you should not try to bend your knee beyond 90° as this may overstrain the joint. Note the caution in Exercise 8.

Good supportive shoes with a cushioned sole will help if you have knee problems. They will absorb some of the jarring that is normally passed on through the knee with every step you take.

Start with 2–4 repetitions of each exercise.

The key knee exercises are 2 and 7.

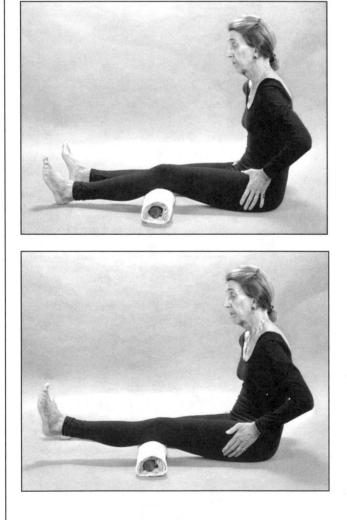

1a. Start: Sit or lie on the floor with your legs out straight. Wrap a rolling pin in a towel. Place it under one leg just above the crease of your knee.

1b. Flex your foot back. Straighten your knee by pushing down onto the towel and lifting your heel. Hold for 3–5 seconds, and then lower slowly.

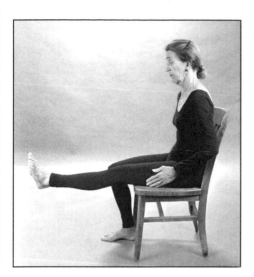

*2. Start: Sit up straight on a chair with your thighs fully supported.

Flex your foot back and straighten your knee. Keep your back straight and your thigh on the chair. Hold for 3–5 seconds, and then lower slowly.

3. Start: Sit up straight about half-way to the edge of the chair.

Extend one foot forward onto its heel and bend the other foot backward onto its toes. Change legs.

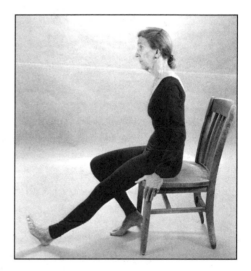

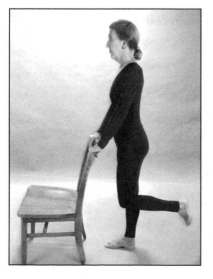

4. Start: Stand, holding the back of a chair with both hands.

Keep your knees together and bend one knee by lifting your foot backward. Lower slowly.

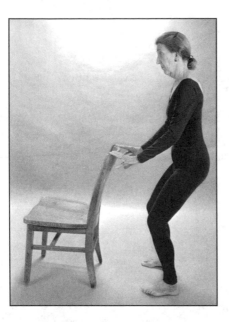

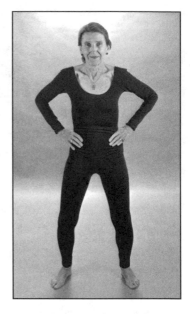

5. Start: Stand with your feet hip-width apart, toes facing forward. Hold the back of a chair for support.

Caution: Take care if you have severe knee problems.

Keep your back straight and slowly bend your knees over your toes. Straighten by pushing up through your feet.

6. Start: Stand with your feet comfortably apart, your toes turned slightly outward. Hold the back of a chair if you need support.

Caution: Take care if you have severe knee problems.

Keep your back straight and slowly bend your knees over your toes. Straighten by pushing up through your feet.

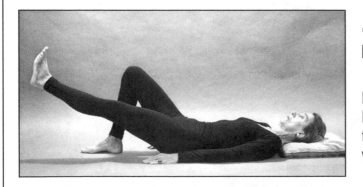

*7. Start: Lie on your back with one leg bent.

Flex back the foot and tighten your knee. Lift your straight leg about 2ft (60 cm) off the floor. Lower slowly, touching the floor with your calf first.

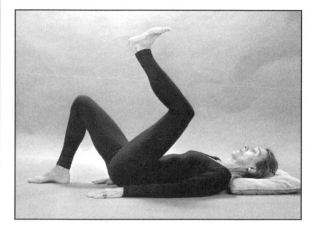

8. Start: Lie on your back with one leg bent.

Caution: Take care with this exercise if you have a hip or knee replacement. Do not bend your hip or knee beyond 90°.

8a. Bend the knee of the straight leg up toward your chest.

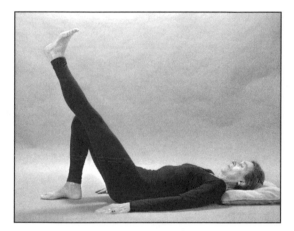

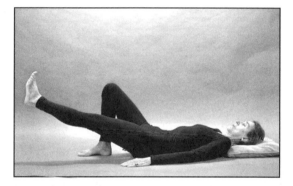

8b–d. Straighten your leg by pushing out with your heel. Bend your leg again, then push out at a different level. Extend at 3–5 different levels.

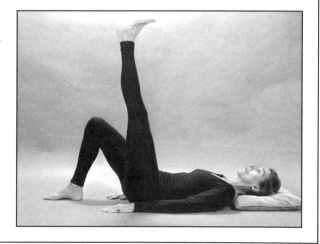

12

Feet

Our feet do so much wonderful work for us—and we so often neglect or abuse them.

The best way to look after your feet is by wearing suitable footwear. Not only will good shoes protect and support them, but they will also cushion your feet and knees to some extent. For everyday wear, choose shoes with rounded toes, a flattish heel and support for the instep. You should be able to move your toes inside your shoes. Another important feature is a shock-absorbing heel and sole. Good-quality jogging shoes are perfect not only for jogging but also for everyday wear—particularly if you spend a lot of time on your feet or like to go walking.

The ankle joint may become inflamed with rheumatoid arthritis or may develop osteoarthritis following a bad ankle injury. Also the ligaments and tendons supporting the joint can easily be sprained. So strengthening the muscles will help support and stabilize the ankle.

The natural arch, or instep, of the foot plays a vital role in keeping us balanced on our feet and in absorbing some of the

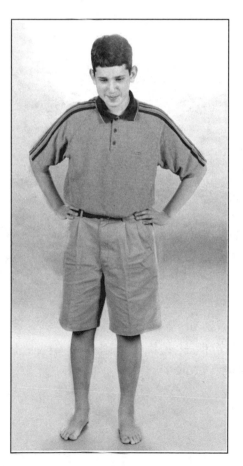

shock of walking. If you have fallen arches, more stress is put onto the bones across the ball of your foot. This can be quite a common site for arthritis. Exercise 4 helps to strengthen the arches of the foot. If your ankles or feet are very painful, do not do the weight-bearing Exercises 6–9.

Start with 2–4 repetitions of each exercise.

The key exercises are 1, 2, and 4.

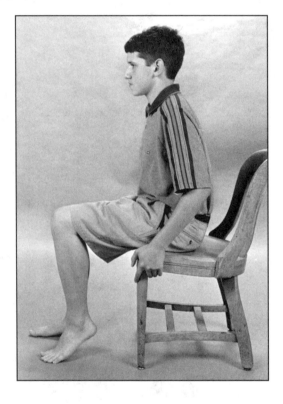 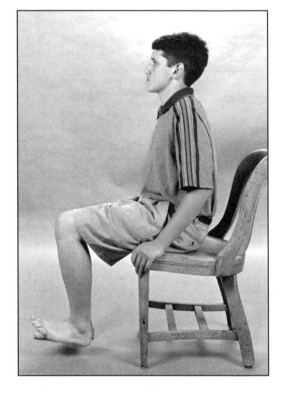

*1. Start: Sit with both feet flat.

1a. Lift the heel of one foot, leaving the ball of your foot on the floor.

1b. Lift up your entire foot by bending it up at the ankle. Lower onto the ball of your foot and then onto your heel. Repeat with the other foot.

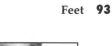
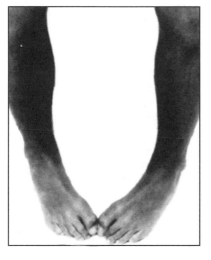

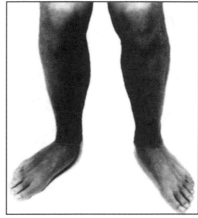

*2. Start: Sit with both feet flat and slightly apart.

2a. Without moving your heels, turn the soles of your feet in toward each other.

2b. Without moving your heels, turn the soles of your feet away from each other.

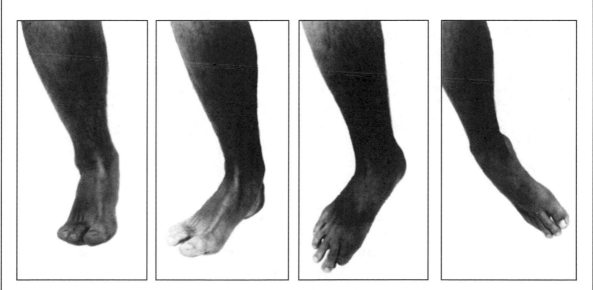

3. Start: Sit with one foot lifted just off the floor.

3a–d. Rotate your foot from the ankle, making a circle with your big toe. Circle the other way.

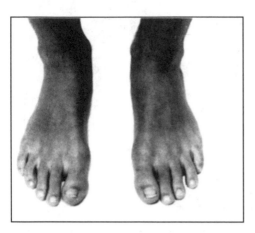

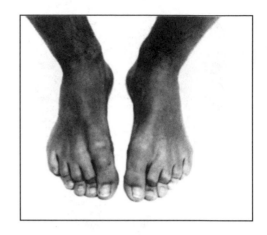

*4a. Start: Sit with your feet flat on the floor.

4b. Keep your heels and toes on the floor and lift the arches on the inside of your feet.

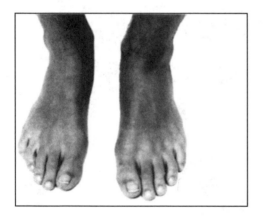

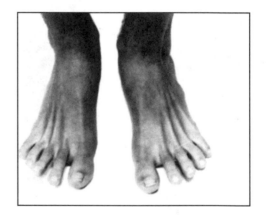

5a. Start: Sit with your feet flat on the floor.

5b. Spread your toes apart and then relax. Keep persevering.

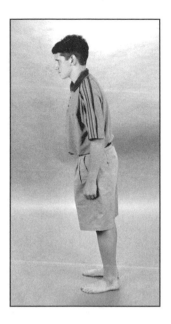 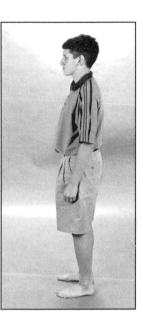

6. Start: Stand up straight with your feet together, toes pointing forward.

6a. Keep your body stiff and your feet flat; sway your weight forward.

6b. Sway your weight backward, keeping your body stiff.

7. Start: Stand with your feet together, holding the back of a chair.

Caution: Take care if you have severe ankle or foot problems.

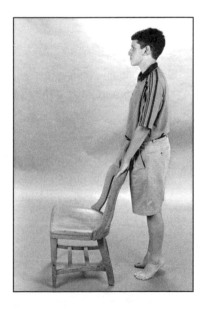 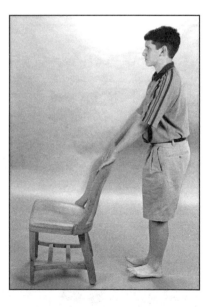

7a. Push up onto your toes.

7b. Lower slowly and then rock back onto your heels and lift your toes.

8. Start: Stand with your feet together, holding the back of a chair.

Caution: Take care if you have severe ankle or foot problems.

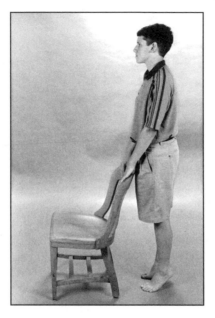 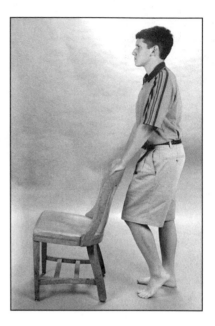

8a. Push up onto your toes.

8b. Slowly lower one heel. Rise up onto your toes again, then lower the other heel.

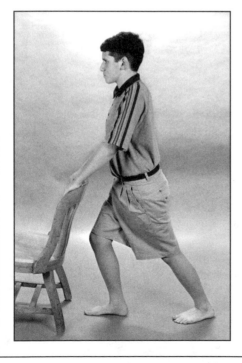

9. Start: Stand with one foot behind the other, both feet facing straight forward. Hold a chair for support.

Keep both heels on the floor as you bend your front knee forward. Keep your back knee straight. Stop when you feel a stretch in the calf of your back leg. Hold the stretch for 3–5 seconds and then slowly release.

Cool-Down

The purpose of the cool-down is to provide a pleasant relaxing completion to your exercise routine. Just as it was necessary to warm up your joints and muscles before doing more strenuous exercises, it is also good to reintegrate your body afterward.

This cool-down exercise combines breathing with movement and should be performed slowly, smoothly, and meditatively. You can sit or stand to do the exercise.

Start by just learning the movement sequence, then begin to combine the breathing with the movements. Once you know what you are doing, think about the quality—let each movement roll smoothly into the next, and feel that each movement "floats" on your breath so that you are moving and breathing together.

This exercise can be done at any time during the day if you are feeling a bit up-tight—its meditative quality will help you to relax.

Repeat the whole sequence 2–4 times.

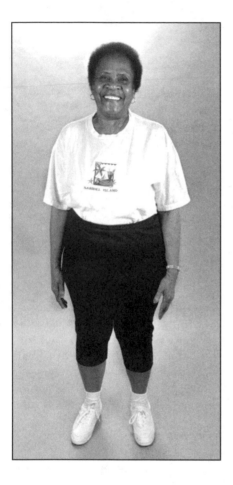

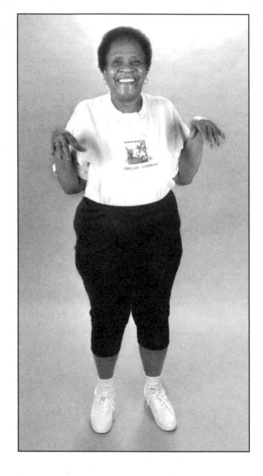

1. Start: Sit or stand with your feet comfortably apart and your arms by your sides. Take a slow breath in and out.

2. Breathe in as you lift your wrists up to your shoulders, keeping your hands relaxed.

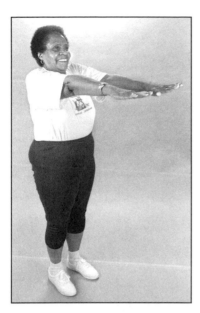

3. Breathe out as you stretch both arms forward, palms down.

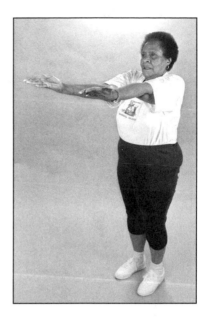

4. Turn your palms upward.

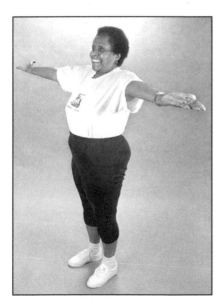

5. Breathe in as you open your arms out to the sides, palms upward.

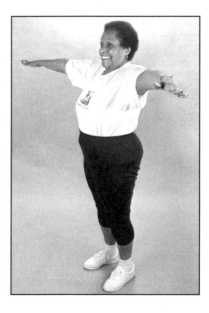

6. Turn your palms down.

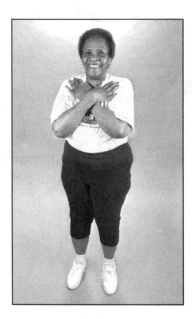

7. Breathe out as you swing your arms down and across your body.

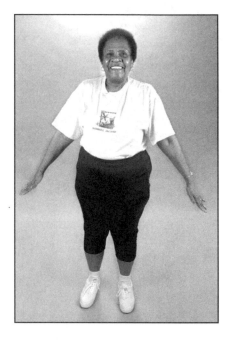

8. Breathe in as you lift your arms out to the side.

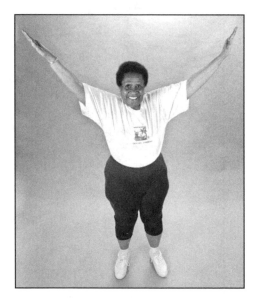

9. Stretch your arms above your head.

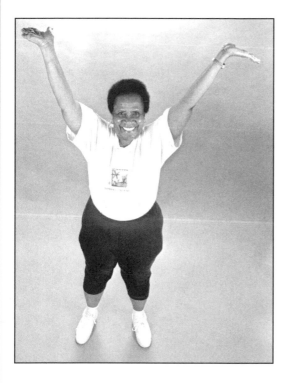

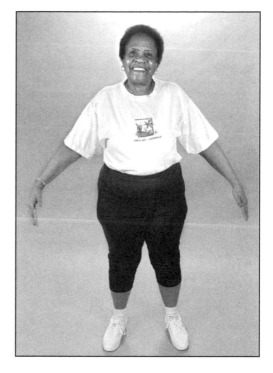

10. Give an extra stretch by pushing upward with the palms of your hands.

11. Breathe out as you lower your arms sideways and return to your starting position.

Repeat movements 1–11 a few times.

Water Exercise

One of the problems of exercising with arthritis is that gravity constantly puts some stress on the joints of the lower body. Not so in the water! The uplifting effect of buoyancy counteracts gravity, so movements that are difficult or impossible on land may be quite feasible and even enjoyable in the water. This is the greatest advantage of water exercise for people with arthritis. As well, water resistance protects the joints from any jarring and provides an easily controlled means of strengthening the

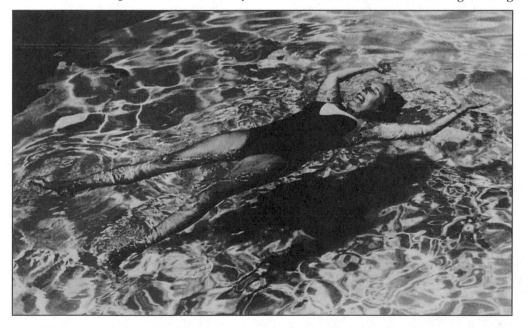

muscles. And, to top it all off, the feeling of weightlessness is wonderfully soothing and relaxing.

Water exercise is not just swimming. It involves using the properties of water to enhance the benefits of exercise. Swimming is an excellent aerobic activity for people with arthritis, but it may not be suitable for everyone, particularly those with back, neck, or shoulder problems. If your pain increases after swimming, choose another form of aerobic exercise such as walking on land or in water, and use the swimming pool for your flexibility and strengthening exercises.

Before you enthusiastically head off to your local swimming pool, take time to check a few details such as water temperature, access in and out of the pool, distance between pool and dressing area, water depth, and, very importantly, quiet and busy periods. Many pools hold aqua-exercise classes, which offer the added pleasure of exercising in a group. Be sure to follow the guidelines on page 32 if you decide to join a class.

Water exercise at home is also possible. You can do leg, foot, hand and finger movements in the bath or put your hands in a basin of warm water to work your fingers. If you have a spa bath, you can also include some arm and leg exercises.

Many people with arthritis are sensitive to the cold, so water temperature can be crucial to the enjoyment of water exercise. A higher temperature is required for gentle exercise than for swimming, so some community pools are not suitable. Ideally, a temperature of 90°–93° Fahrenheit (32°–34° Celsius) is preferred for gentle exercise—particularly by those who are cold-sensitive. For swimming or more vigorous exercise, a lower temperature is more comfortable. There are some special hydrotherapy pools,

but these are not always available to the general public. Maybe you could take the opportunity to lobby your park board commissioner or fitness center about the needs of the many people with arthritis!

Water depth is also important. The joint being exercised needs to be under the water so it enjoys the full advantages provided by buoyancy and warmth. However, don't go above armpit level, or you will start to float away! The most stable position in the water is squatting with your feet wide apart, knees bent, and head forward. This way you are well balanced and still have your shoulders under the water.

Perhaps it has been quite some time since you have been in the water. Until you regain your confidence, find a time when the pool is not full of exuberant children and go with someone who can give you support if necessary. For the first time, maybe just walk around and get the feel of the water and the effect of buoyancy.

Many people find that exercise in water seems less strenuous than on land. Certainly the support provided by the water does encourage freedom of movement. Because of this ease of movement, it is tempting to do too much. You will soon realize that a water exercise session works your joints and muscles quite strongly and moves them in unaccustomed ways. As with all forms of exercise, if your pain level increases markedly, you should exercise more gently next time. Be assured that in the water you won't have done any damage. People often feel quite tired after a water exercise session due to the combination of exercise and warm water. If this is your experience, have a rest afterward or, better still, do one of the relaxation exercises.

The exercises described in the following pages give a good range of general movements for the whole body. You can also add many of the exercises described in the other sections of the book. Remember, if you are adapting a land exercise for the water, the moving joint should remain under the water. Some suitable exercises to do in the water are:

Neck: 3, 4, 5, 6

Arms: 3, 4, 5

Hands: 1, 2, 3, 4, 5, 6

Back: 7, 9

Hips: 3, 4

Knees: 4, 5, 6

Feet: 2, 3, 4, 5, 7, 8, 9

Cool-down: Let your arms float through the water.

It is simple to regulate how much effort you use in the water. You can make an exercise work you harder either by moving faster or by pushing through the water with a broad surface, such as the palm of your hand or a flat piece of apparatus.

Some of the movements use flotation equipment. It can be bought, but the cheapest, simplest float is an empty plastic bottle. The larger the bottle, the greater the resistance it will supply, so experiment and choose a size that suits your capabilities.

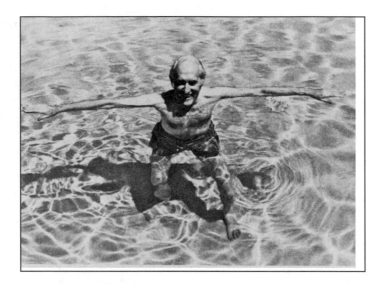

1. Start: Stand with feet apart and shoulders under water.

1a. Allow the buoyancy of the water to lift your arms out sideways.

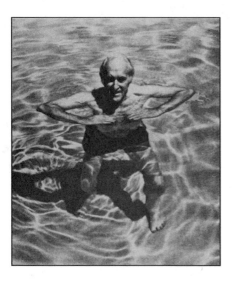

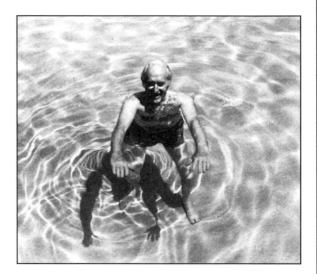

1b. Rest your arms on the surface of the water and bend your elbows.

1c. Stretch forward with both hands. Lower your arms by pushing gently down through the water. Repeat the movement in the opposite direction—float arms up in front, bring hands to shoulders, open out sideways, and push down to the side of your body.

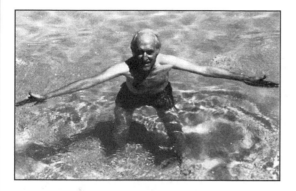

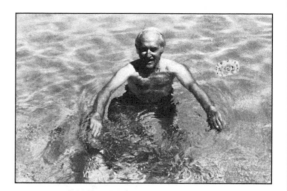

2. Start: Stand with shoulders underwater, arms out to the side with palms facing forward.

2a. Push through the surface of the water, bringing your palms together in front of your chest.

2b. Turn your palms outward and push out and back through the water.

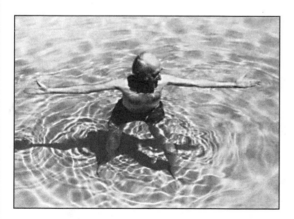

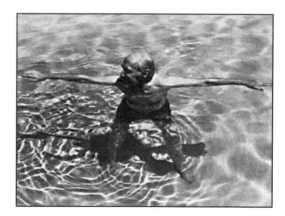

3. Start: Stand with shoulders underwater and arms floating out to the side.

3a. Turn your head to one side and twist your arms so your palms face upward.

3b. Turn your head to the other side as you twist your palms down and back.

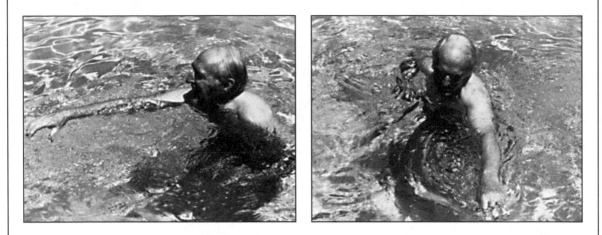

4. Start: Stand in a stable position with feet apart and shoulders underwater.

4a. Reach out with alternate hands and grab at the water.

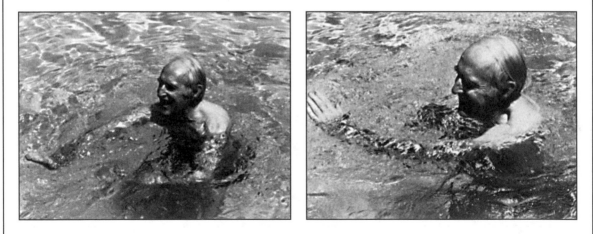

4b. Push outward through the water in all directions with the palms of your hands.

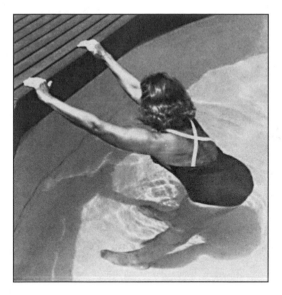

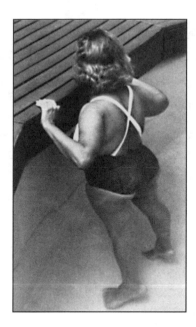

5. Start: Stand close to the side of the pool, holding the edge or a rail with both hands.

5a. Gently stretch backward with your bottom.

5b. Straighten your body and bring your stomach toward the side of the pool, so you <u>gently</u> arch your lower back. Continue to swing easily and gently forward and backward.

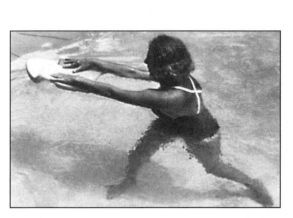

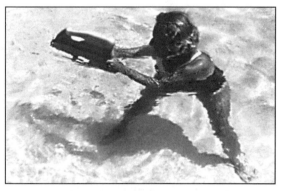

6. Stand in a stable position, with your feet apart and shoulders underwater holding a kickboard or other float.

6a. Rest your hands on the float and swing it gently from side to side. Keep your feet flat and twist from the waist.

6b. Hold the float vertically and push it through the water from one side to the other. Keep your legs and pelvis still and twist from the waist.

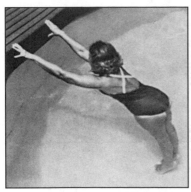 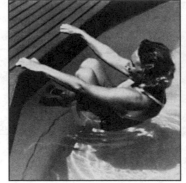 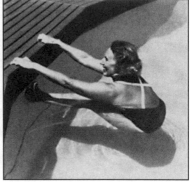

7. Start: Stand close to the side of the pool, holding the edge or rail with both hands.

7a. Walk back with both feet as far as possible.

7b. Walk into the side and up the wall with your knees bent.

7c. Gently straighten your legs and stretch backward.

Caution: Do not walk up the side of the pool if you have a hip replacement.

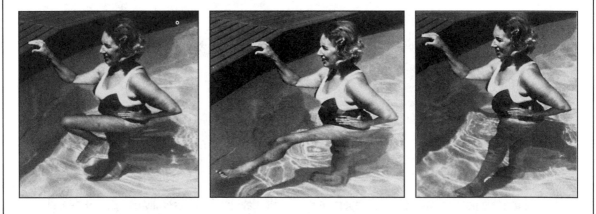

8. Start: Stand close to the edge of the pool, holding the side with one hand. Work your outside leg.

8a,b,c. Bend at the hip and knee to make large circles with your foot, as though you are pedaling a bicycle. Turn around to work your other leg.

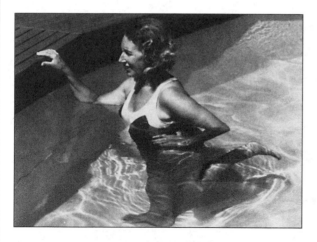

9. Start: Stand close to the edge of the pool, holding the side with one hand. Work your outside leg.

9a. Bend one leg and lift your foot backward.

9b. Straighten your leg and kick forward.

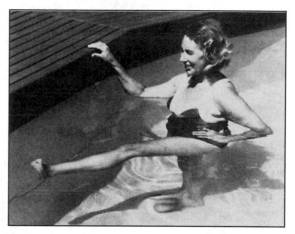

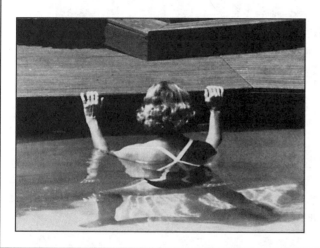

10. Start: Stand holding the side of the pool, with both hands and feet spread as far apart as comfortable. Keep your feet flat and your knees over your toes, and lunge gently from side to side.

11. Start: Stand in water at waist to mid-chest depth.

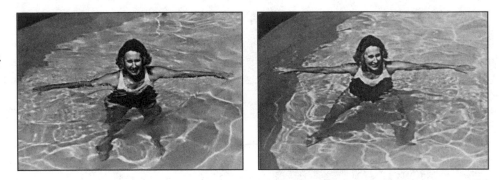

11a,b. Step sideways for four short steps, then four long steps. Repeat in the other direction.

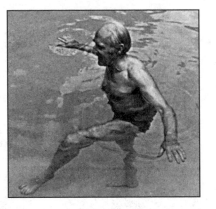
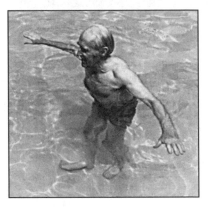

11c,d. Walk four steps forward lifting your knees. Walk four steps backward on your heels.

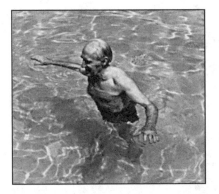
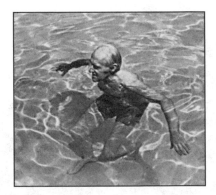

11e,f. Walk four steps forward on your toes. Walk four steps forward with your knees bent and your shoulders underwater.

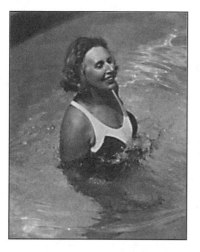

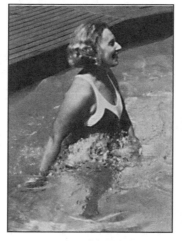

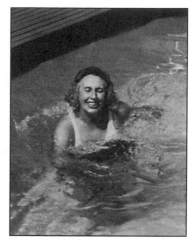

12. Start: Stand in water at about mid-chest depth. Hold the edge if necessary.

12a. Jog gently on the spot, lifting your knees.

12b,c. Jump and twist your body from side to side.

Caution: Take care you do not overstress any arthritic joints in your back, hips, knees, or feet. Move to deeper water or hold onto the edge to lessen the impact.

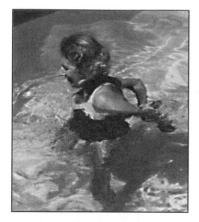

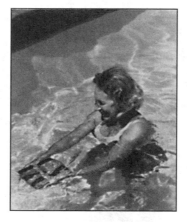

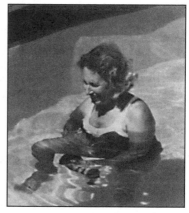

13. Start: Stand in water at about mid-chest level, with a ball or other small float.

13a,b. Keep the float under the water and pass it behind your back and in front of your body. Pass it around in the reverse direction.

13c. Pass the float under alternate legs.

Aerobic Exercise

The value of aerobic or endurance exercise in your overall exercise program has already been mentioned. Until fairly recently, the more strenuous activities and sports have usually been considered inappropriate for most people with arthritis. Suitable exercise was limited to the therapeutic regime prescribed by a doctor or physical therapist. This form of exercise is certainly important in the management of arthritis, but many studies are now showing that the more strenuous fitness activities are also appropriate and beneficial, provided the arthritis is under control.

The term *aerobic* means *living with air*. When applied to exercise, it signifies you are able to breathe normally while doing the activity. This implies a moderate level of exertion. Of course, your breathing will be deeper and fuller, but if you start to become very puffed you are working beyond your aerobic capacity.

During aerobic exercise your heart and lungs have to work harder so that more oxygen-containing blood is circulated to the working muscles. You breathe a bit harder, and your heart rate is increased. Regular aerobic exercise increases the efficiency and capacity of your lungs, your heart, and the rest of your circulatory system and has a beneficial effect on your whole body. Also, it is the form of exercise that helps with weight reduction since it increases the body's energy consumption—provided you don't increase your level of food consumption!

To gain maximum advantage from aerobic exercise, it is recommended that you

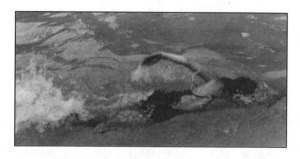

exercise large muscle groups at a moderate intensity for a 20–30 minute session, three or four times per week. Longer, harder, and more often does not dramatically increase the benefits, and it may lead to injury. Although this is what you might aim for, do not try to start there if you are unused to exercise. Begin with shorter, easier sessions and build up gradually and steadily. By pushing yourself to pain and exhaustion you will only defeat the whole purpose of what you are attempting to achieve.

Getting Started

It is a good idea to check with your doctor before you start your aerobic program. This is absolutely essential if you have:

- Moderate to severe arthritis

- A heart condition

- High blood pressure

- A history of chest pains, fainting spells, or severe dizziness

- Any other medical condition that may affect your exercise capacity

Now choose one or two activities you like and in which you can participate without overstressing your arthritic joints. Some suitable activities might be walking, swimming, cycling, dancing, table tennis, golf, stair-climbing, low-impact exercise-to-music or aquarobics classes, water exercises, and lawn-mowing—anything that can be maintained for about 20–30 minutes at a fairly constant level of moderate exertion.

Of course, you do not have to commence with a 20-minute session. Start where you are now. You will be amazed at how you can build this up gradually and steadily over a period of time.

Having chosen your activity, determine what you can do easily. Rather than trying to maintain a constant level of exertion, you might like to alternate periods of activity with rest intervals. For instance, if you decide to take up walking, try walking briskly for three minutes and slowly for one minute. Maintain this pattern for 10 minutes or so. Or you could climb one flight of stairs at a time with a 30-second rest in between. Remember, you are aiming for a moderate level of exertion over an extended period.

Determining Exercise Intensity

The measure of exercise intensity is not what you are doing, but how hard you are doing it. An easy way of regulating your exercise intensity is the "talk test." Moderate exertion should allow you to talk or sing comfortably. If you are too short of breath to do this, you are working too hard.

Some people prefer a more scientific approach. By taking note of your pulse rate during the activity, you will have a good idea how hard your heart is working. Note that this test is not suitable for someone on medication to regulate heart rate.

At rest, your heart beats at a certain rate, normally about 65–75 beats per minute. With exercise and other forms of stimulation, heart rate increases. Everyone has a maximum rate at which their heart can beat. To be effective, aerobic exercise should increase your heart rate to 60–80 percent of its maximum. This is your target heart rate. It is age-related, so use the following table as an indication of what you should aim for:

Age	Target pulse rate (per minute)
20–30	117–156
30–40	111–148
40–50	105–140
50–60	99–132
60–70	93–124
70–80	87–116
80+	84–112

Aim to work with your pulse rate between these two levels. Slow down if you are above the upper level, and gradually increase your exercise intensity if you are below the lower level. When you first start, take your pulse a few times during your exercise session and then retest whenever you make any changes.

Building Up

There are three ways to increase your level of aerobic exercise: by distance, time, and weight. Aim at increasing only one factor at a time. Always maintain the same level for at least 10–14 days, three times per week, before contemplating any further increases. These should be made in small increments. Do not add more than one quarter of what you are doing at present. Continue at this level for another 10-14 days.

Extra distance can be covered by increasing intensity or by exercising for a longer period. Another way of using time to add to your activity level is by gradually reducing rest intervals. The addition of weight (not body weight, of course!) will also increase your level of exertion. When walking or stair-climbing you can carry small weights or wear a back-pack. Wearing a T-shirt or extra bathing costume achieves the same effect in the water.

Warming Up and Cooling Down

As with other forms of exercise, take time warming up your muscles and joints and gradually increasing your heart rate before you exert yourself fully. Likewise, allow your body to slowly relax and return to a less active state afterward.

The Warm-Up and Cool-Down sections in this book are suitable for this purpose. You might like to add some of your other flexibility and strengthening exercises as well. After aerobic exercise your whole body is well warmed, and this is an ideal time to include some flexibility exercises. Another method of warming up and cooling down is to start and end your aerobic session with just a few minutes at a more gentle pace.

Specific Aerobic Activities

Walking

This is by far the easiest and most common form of exercise. The advantages of walking are many. It is a wonderful exercise for strengthening the heart, lungs, bones, hips, and knees. It is also easy, inexpensive, convenient, sociable, and safe. Make sure you wear well-fitting, supportive shoes with nonslippery, shock-absorbing soles. Choose a suitable area in which to walk, avoiding hills, uneven surfaces, soft ground, and gravel. If the weather is a bit inclement, you can always walk around an indoor shopping center.

Swimming and Water Exercise

The many advantages and benefits of water activities for people with arthritis are described elsewhere (page 103).

Bicycling

Riding a bicycle can be a very enjoyable way of exercising. It is best if you can cycle in a fairly flat area away from the hazards of heavy traffic. A new bicycle can be quite expensive, so first determine whether you like this form of exercise and then buy one that suits your requirements.

Stationary bicycles (exercise bikes) avoid the problems of balance, safety, and inconvenience. Try to borrow or hire a stationary bicycle before you go to the expense of buying one. Many people appreciate the convenience. They cope with the boredom of sitting in one place by watching television or listening to the radio or music.

Stair-Climbing

This is not such a good option if you have problems with your hips or knees, but it is convenient and can easily be fitted into a work routine. Think of using the stairs rather than the elevator.

Exercise-to-Music Classes

Many places conduct regular low-impact aerobic classes. These classes have no running or jumping, but they can be quite strenuous and so may put strain on the joints. Some classes are designed for older adults; these are gentler and thus more suitable. Before starting, go along and observe a class. Points to check are whether there is a warm-up and a cool-down period, the overall intensity of the session, the amount of strain being put on the joints, the general attitude of the class, and whether the instructor is encouraging participants to work at their own pace. If you decide to join, tell the instructor you have arthritis, and he or she may be able to give you some advice on adapting certain exercises. Remember the guidelines about safe exercise practices and follow them, even if this means you cannot always keep up with the rest of the class.

Other Activities

There are many sports and activities, such as dancing, table tennis, tennis, golf, and tai chi, that can provide safe, enjoyable exercise for someone with arthritis. Which is most suitable for you depends on your own preference and how it affects your arthritic joints. Don't be afraid to try something new. Just take it easy at first and monitor your own pain level.

Exercise Opportunities

As exercise is becoming more and more popular in the community, there are increasing opportunities to engage in a variety of activities. Some places to try for ideas are:

Arthritis Foundation

Community health centers

Community centers

Adult education courses

Senior citizens clubs

Recreation and leisure centers

Health and fitness clubs and gymnasiums

Local newspaper

Local swimming pool

YWCA and YMCA

16

Relaxation

For some of us, relaxation is the most difficult exercise of all. It is easy to say to someone else, "Don't worry about it. Just relax." But when we are dealing with our own pain or our own problems and worries, it's a different matter. We find that relaxation does not always come easily.

Whether you have arthritis or not, relaxation is one of the most important exercises you can ever learn. If you do have arthritis, you are no doubt aware that it causes you more trouble when you are upset or under stress. It may seem that you experience more pain, or maybe it's just that you are less able to cope with it.

The connection also works the other way. Prolonged pain can be very depressing and often creates inner tension. With arthritis also, the muscles surrounding a joint may tense up to prevent any movement that may cause

pain. This close interaction between pain and tension can result in a downward spiral in which pain causes tension . . . causes more pain . . . causes more tension . . . and so on!

If you want to start coming up again, you have to break the cycle by reducing either your pain or your tension. We know pain can be relieved by the use of comfort techniques (refer to page 20) or by appropriate medication. But relaxation is very helpful in reducing your general level of tension, both physical and mental. By lessening your general tension, you are able to cope much better with your level of pain.

There are a number of techniques you can use to develop a sense of deep relaxation. We will describe some of these. Remember, though, that relaxation is like any other skill. Practice is the key to success. This means that you should do these exercises regularly, not just when you are feeling uptight.

Relaxation is a natural complement to physical activity. Regular physical exercise works the muscles of the body and so helps to release general muscle tension. A good time to practice your relaxation is just after you have completed your workout.

Methods of Relaxation

First, a number of quick and easy ways to relax—yawning, laughing, sighing, stretching, or shaking various parts or all your body, and doing the cool-down exercise (page 97).

Certain activities that don't require a lot of concentration can be very relaxing. Perhaps you enjoy reading, knitting, walking along the beach, listening to music, or working in the garden.

You might like to relieve your muscle tension by soaking in a hot bath or spa or by treating yourself to a massage. What bliss!

All these suggestions are useful; but a deeper form of relaxation, which quiets your mind as well as releasing tension from your body, is more beneficial. You need about 15–20 minutes in which to practice these deep relaxation techniques, so choose a time when you will be undisturbed.

We have included a number of different techniques for you to try. You will find that some work for you better than others. Try them all, and then choose the methods you find most beneficial.

For the first few sessions, you may not achieve deep relaxation. You may think you have failed to do the exercise correctly. But if you are very tense or in a lot of pain, it's more difficult to achieve a deep level of relaxation. The more you practice, the easier it gets.

It is well worth persevering because it's in these situations that you have most need of relaxation. What you must remember is

not to try too hard. Relaxation will come of its own accord if you can adopt a passive attitude without too many expectations.

Relaxation Positions

Before you start, make sure your body is comfortable and fully supported. It is best to lie on the floor or a firm bed with a low pillow for your head. A chair is all right provided it gives your body good support, preferably with a head rest.

Three lying positions are shown. Try these or find another position in which you feel comfortable. Keep warm throughout your relaxation session. As your body becomes more relaxed it cools down, so cover yourself with a light blanket, particularly if you have been exercising. Be sure that your clothing is not restrictive. Loosen anything that is tight around your body. Take off your shoes.

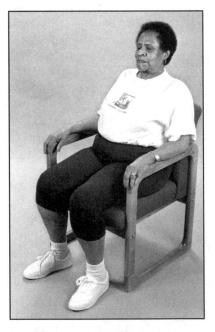

Sit well back into a chair with your thighs supported and your feet flat on the floor.

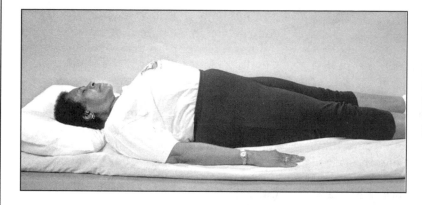

Lie on your back with a low pillow under your head. Have your legs slightly apart and let your feet fall outward. Rest your arms by your sides.

Lie on your back with a low pillow under your head. Bend up both legs so your feet are comfortably apart and your knees rest together. This is a good position if you have low back pain.

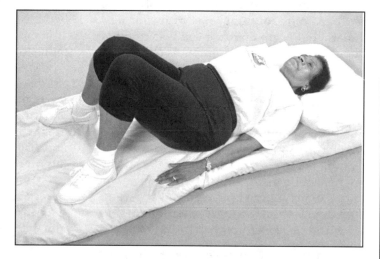

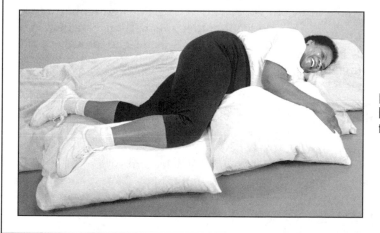

Lie on your side with a low pillow under your head. Rest your top arm and leg forward on two pillows.

Technique 1: Concentration on Breathing

Lie down in your comfortable supported position. As you lie there, become aware of your breath. Follow the air as you breathe in and breathe out. Allow your breath to flow easily and evenly. Don't try to force yourself to take deep breaths. After a short time, start to count each breath silently as you breathe out. Begin with the first breath out as "one" and continue up to "ten." Then start again at "one." If you find yourself drifting off into other thoughts, don't worry. Just start again by counting 'one' with your next breath. It doesn't matter if you lose count or repeat numbers. The counting is only a way of focusing your mind. It's not significant in itself.

Keep concentrating on your breathing for about 10–15 minutes. You can open your eyes occasionally to look at the clock, but position it so that you don't have to move your head. Experience and enjoy the feeling of relaxation for a short time before you think about getting up. When you are ready, move and stretch a little, then open your eyes and *slowly* sit up.

Technique 2: Breathing into Various Parts of the Body

Settle into a comfortable position and then concentrate on your breath. Allow it to flow evenly and rhythmically, without force. Concentrate on your *out-breath*. Imagine that with each breath out you are releasing stored-up tensions from your body. Don't think about the in-breath. It will take care of itself.

After about 10 of these breaths, imagine that you are breathing out through various parts of your body. As your breath flows through, it releases the tension from that part of your body. Imagine breathing out through your right leg . . . your left leg . . . your pelvic area . . . your stomach . . . your right arm . . . your left arm . . . between your shoulder blades . . . down your back . . . over your face . . . and through your hair. Send two or three breaths to each body region and then spend some time on your problem area. Imagine that your breath is warm and soothing. Imagine that, as it flows through your arthritic joints, it relieves the pain and releases the tension in the surrounding muscles.

Finish by enjoying the sense of peace and relaxation you have produced in your body. Gradually come back by moving and stretching a little, opening your eyes, and then slowly getting up.

These are just a few ways in which you can learn to experience relaxation. You can learn other relaxation techniques at yoga and meditation classes or stress management courses. There are books you can read and also some relaxation tapes available that talk you through your relaxation session.

Try to practice relaxation three or four times each week. After a while the feeling of deep relaxation comes much more easily. You will soon discover that you can use the techniques effectively when you are tense or in pain. Perhaps it will dawn on you that you are generally less tense and better able to cope with your pain. Remember, relaxation is another means that can help you manage your arthritis. The power of the mind is very strong. Regular deep relaxation can reduce or replace your reliance on pain medication.

Relaxation and Sleep

Maybe you fell asleep during or after a relaxation session. That's fine. It means you were truly relaxed. If you do not sleep well during the night, this is a good opportunity to catch up on some sleep. Painful joints often make undisturbed sleep difficult if you have arthritis. By resting and sleeping for a while during the day, you'll need less sleep during the night.

General tiredness is a common problem for people with arthritis, particularly rheumatoid arthritis. If you do get weary during the day, listen to your body. Plan your daily activities so that you can have a half-hour to one-hour rest period. This may make the difference between coping and not coping with the rest of the day.

You can try these techniques at night if you have difficulty getting off to sleep or if you wake up through the night. In this situation the same thoughts may keep circling around and around in your head. You need to break this cycle by focusing your thoughts in a different direction. All the techniques described above can be useful in refocusing and quietening your thoughts. Select the technique with which you are most comfortable. Try it the next time you are having trouble finding those sweet dreams.

17

Using Your Body

Arthritis affects the way you use your body. Obviously pain, weakness, stiffness, and lack of mobility will make movement difficult. However, this does not have to prevent you from doing what you want. Some of the factors contributing to poor movement can be improved. By starting an exercise program as described in this book you are already doing much toward this end. And there are some other methods that might also help.

Look at young children and notice how freely and easily they move. As adults, some people seem to have maintained this ability to move gracefully without any apparent effort. Others are stiff, awkward, and full of tension. It is this tension that is the key. Our muscles gradually accumulate evidence of the physical and psychological stresses of our lives. Rather than moving freely, we tend to hold on to ourselves with unneces-

sary muscle tension and to fix our movements into habitual patterns.

There are many simple, everyday activities that use far more energy than required. For instance, do you need to have your jaw clenched tight or your shoulders up near your ears in order to read this page? You will find that, as you practice the relaxation exercises in the previous chapter, you will become more and more aware of any unnecessary muscle tension and eventually you will develop the ability to release it at will.

In some of the common everyday postures and movements, such as standing, sitting, standing up, and lifting, we have developed habitual ways of moving that are very inefficient and actually put extra strain on the joints. It is not easy to change these movement patterns because anything else will not feel "right". But if you recognize that the new ways are better for your body, your perseverance will pay off. You can develop a different, less stressful way.

Posture

Were you often told to sit up straight? Well, good posture not only makes you look better, but it also puts less strain on your joints. Maintaining good posture does not just mean standing or sitting in the "correct" position. Posture is a dynamic activity, so you need to be just as aware of it when you are moving as when you are still.

Have you noticed what happens to your posture when you are feeling "on top of the world" compared to when you are feeling "down in the dumps"? Our emotions are expressed in the way we sit, stand, and move. It can work the other way too. By lifting your body, you help to lift your spirits.

Of course, it's a lot easier to sag and slump rather than make the effort to maintain good posture. But have you forgotten that one of the functions of muscles is to take some of the strain off the joints? By slouching, you are hanging the weight of your body onto the ligaments and other structures surrounding the joints. This can put extra stress on an already damaged joint. But the other extreme is just about as bad—using a lot of muscular effort trying to hold a straight rigid posture. This will just make your joints feel stiffer.

Good posture comes from a dynamic balance of muscular forces. It essentially relies on good tone in the postural muscles. As you continue with your exercise pro-

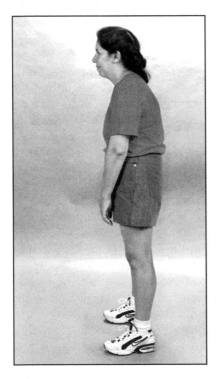

Bad posture

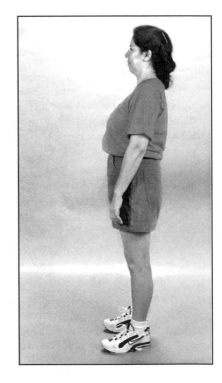

Good posture

gram, you will find that your posture improves automatically.

The best way to align your body correctly is to imagine that the crown of your head is attached by a string to a balloon and that the rest of your body is suspended from it. Think of being lifted up through the central axis of your body. When you apply this concept, you will find that your back and neck lengthen and straighten, your shoulders drop and fall back, your chest lifts, your tummy flattens, and your buttocks tuck under. Just be sure you have not also lifted your chin or shoulders. Your shoulders contribute nothing to the lengthening of your spine, and your chin should remain slightly dropped because you are lifting through the *crown* of your head (refer to Neck Exercise 2, page 51).

Look at yourself in a mirror and see the difference. But be conscious that this is not a static position. Try to think of that balloon when you are walking or doing your exercises, and throughout all your other daily activities.

Sitting posture is important, too. We spend so much of our life in chairs. Many modern chairs seem to encourage us to sink into them, and it is virtually impossible to maintain a good sitting posture. Not only are they difficult to get out of, but often they do not give very good support to your body and soon become quite uncomfortable.

The ideal comfortable chair allows you to sit with your bottom back in the chair—your thighs fully supported and your feet flat on the floor. The back of the chair

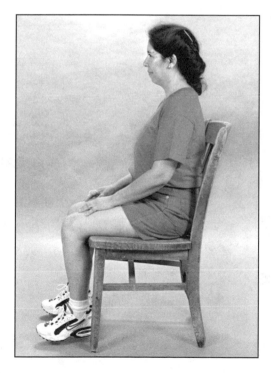

Good posture

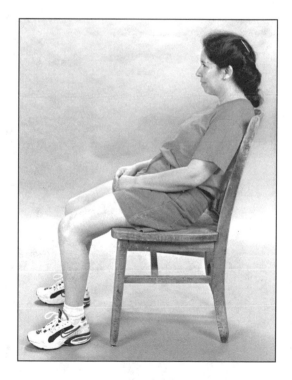

Bad posture

should offer firm support right along your spine. It is useful to have arm rests.

Of course, you can still think of the balloon holding you up when you are sitting. Slumping in a chair will eventually lead to low back ache because of the strain being put on the ligaments and muscles of the lumbar spine. A small cushion placed behind your lower back often relieves back ache. This is a particularly useful item for long car journeys since many car seats are not very supportive.

Key exercises for posture:

Warm-Up 5

Neck 2, 6

Back 1, 6, 7, 8

Feet 6

Getting Up from a Chair

You know by now that sitting for too long only leads to your becoming stiffer and even less interested in getting up. It is no wonder that many people prefer to remain sitting when they realize what a struggle it can be to lift their body weight up against gravity—especially with pain and weakness in hips and knees. But there is a way of getting up more easily by using the principle of momentum.

The first trick is to sit in a decent chair, as described before. Low-level lounge chairs require an ejector seat! Now, try the following method:

1. Move forward to the edge of the seat.

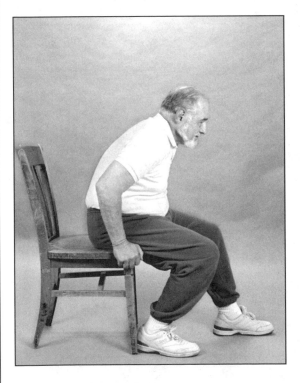

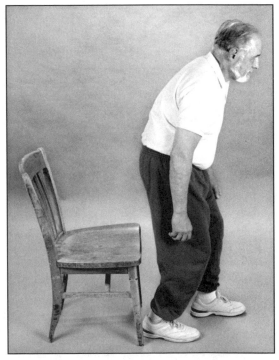

2. Place both feet on the floor about hip-width apart. They can be parallel or with one foot in front of the other, depending on the site of your arthritis. Experiment to find what is most comfortable for you.

3. Bend forward from the hips (not the waist). This is the same movement as Back Exercise 1. In fact, do this movement a few times.

4. As you rock forward, let the momentum of the movement carry you *forward and up* into standing. The farther you rock forward, the easier it is to rise.

5. Sitting down is just the reverse of this procedure. Position yourself back against the chair, then release the hip and knee joints so your bottom goes back and down onto the seat and your nose heads toward your knees.

Lifting

Lifting incorrectly puts a great strain on your lower back. Do not bend over when you want to lift something up from the floor or ground, or take something out from a low cupboard or shelf. Instead, you should use the strong muscles of your legs to do the work.

So, when lifting, always try to follow this sequence:

1. Bend your knees and squat down close to the object you want to lift.

2. Lift the object and hold it close to your body.

3. Keep your *back straight* and stand up by *straightening your knees.*

The only problem with this method is that it does put a strain on your knees. If you have pain in your knee, use your mouth

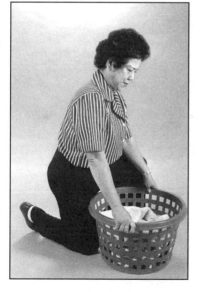
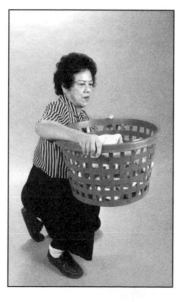
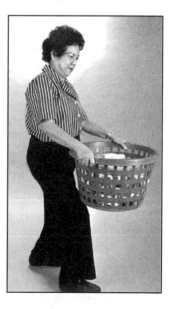

Lifting

to lift heavy objects—ask someone else! You don't want to have an injured back as well as a bad knee!

Getting Down to and Up from the Floor

Many people rule out exercises or relaxation on the floor because of the difficulty and potential danger of getting down and up again. The following method is safe and does not require a lot of effort.

Getting Down

1. Position a chair with floor space in front of it. Sit on it with feet well apart.
2. Hold the seat with one hand and slide forward and sideways off it so you are kneeling with one knee up (same side as supporting hand) and one knee down.
3. Kneel onto both hands and knees. Your arthritis will determine which is the best order for you to bear weight on your hands and knees.
4. Bend one elbow and lower your body onto its side.
5. It is easy now to lie over onto your back.

Getting Up

Reverse the above procedure.

1. Bend both knees and roll onto your side and up onto all fours.
2. Adjust your position so you are now kneeling in front of the chair.
3. Use the chair for support and come into a half-kneeling position, lifting the knee closest the chair.
4. Push up with your hand and swivel so you can place your bottom on the seat.

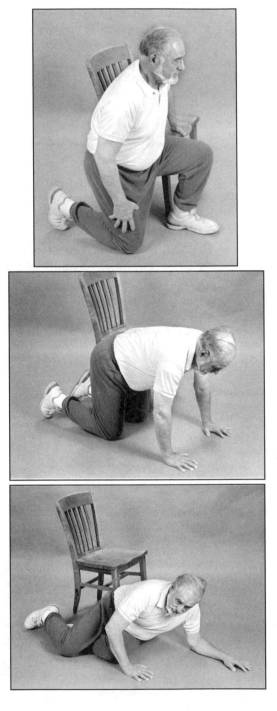

Getting down onto the floor

Obviously this method is not suitable for everyone with arthritis. It does put some strain on the hips, knees, shoulders, and hands. You may find that you can go one way in step 1, but not the other. If you have any doubts about your ability to cope with this procedure, make sure you have someone nearby for assistance.

Everyday Efficiency

Here are a few more pointers on how to make life easier for yourself and less stressful on your joints.

- Determine your priorities—some tasks are not really necessary.
- Before you do anything, think: "What is the easiest way of doing this task?"

- Ask for help to do tasks that might overstress your joints.
- Organize work areas so items you want to use are within easy reach.
- Plan your work tasks and work space so you can function efficiently.
- Balance work and rest by scheduling frequent, short rest periods throughout the day.
- Use mechanical aids and devices that reduce stress on your joints.
- For further advice in this area consult an occupational therapist.

Index

Abdominal muscles. *See* Stomach muscles
Aerobic exercises, 24, 115–118
  benefits of, 115–116
  classes for, 118
  intensity of, 116–117
  types of, 116, 117–118
Aging, and arthritis, 5
Ankles
  arthritis in, 91
  exercises for, 35, 47
Ankylosing spondylitis, 7
  back exercises for, 66, 76–77
Anti-inflammatory drugs, 19
Antimalarial drugs, 19
Arms
  arthritis in, 53
  exercises for, 37, 39, 48, 54–58, 106–108, 113
  pain and numbness in, 49
Arthritis
  and aerobic exercise, 115–116
  and aging, 5
  ankylosing spondylitis, 7
  bursitis, 7–8
  comfort techniques for, 20
  common sites of, 3, 4, 5–6, 7, 9
  definition of, 1, 15
  and diet, 15–17
  and doctor appointments, 17–18
  effects of, on joints, 1–2
  and exercise, 4, 6–7, 10, 12, 23–32
  fibromyalgia, 9–10
  and immune system, 3–4
  and medication, 18–19
  and mental attitude, 17
  and movement, 125–131
  osteoarthritis, 4–7
  vs. osteoporosis, 10–13
  rheumatoid, 2–4, 8, 25
  risk factors for, 5, 8, 11
  and stress, 17
  surgery for, 20
  symptoms of, 1, 4, 5, 7, 8, 9
  tendonitis, 7–8
  treatments for, 4, 6–7, 8, 9, 18–19
  types of, 2–11
  weather and, 21
Arthritis Foundation, 21
Artificial joints, 20
Aspirin, 19

Back
  ankylosing spondylitis in, 66
  arthritis in, 5, 7–8, 65–66
  exercises for, 36, 37, 46, 47, 67–77, 109

Bed, getting out of, 35, 40–41
Bicycling, 118
Blood vessels, and rheumatoid arthritis, 4
Bones
  changes in density of, 11
  in joints, 1
  and osteoporosis, 10–12
Breathing, 27
  exercises for, 34, 44, 122
Bursae, 2
  and bursitis, 9
Bursitis, 8–9

Calf muscles, 96
Cartilage, in joints, 2, 6
Cervical spondylosis.
  See Osteoarthritis
Chest pain, and aerobic exercise, 116
Circulation, 43–44
Clothing
  for exercise, 24–25, 26
  for warmth, 20
Contact sports, 24
Cool-down exercises, 97–101, 117
Corticosteroids, 19
Cortisone, 19

Degenerative joint disease.
  See Osteoarthritis
DEXA (dual energy X-ray absorptiometry) scan, 12
Diet, 15–17
Dizziness, and aerobic exercise, 116
Doctor appointments, 17–18

Efficiency, pointers for, 131
Elbows
  arthritis in, 53
  bursitis in, 9
  exercises for, 45, 55–58
  tendonitis in, 9
Endurance exercises. *See* Aerobic exercises
Exercise, 23–32
  aerobic, 24, 115–118
  and ankylosing spondylitis, 7
  clothing for, 26
  and fibromyalgia, 10
  and osteoarthritis, 5–6
  and osteoporosis, 12
  and inflamed joints, 25
  length of time required for, 26
  and medication, 26
  and motivation, 30–32
  pain after, 25, 27
  places to, 26

planning program of, 27–29
  reasons for, 23–24
  and relaxation, 27, 119–123
  and rheumatoid arthritis, 4, 25
  time of day to, 26
  tips for, 24–27, 29, 30–32
  types of, 24
  warm-up, 26, 44–48
  what body parts to, 25–26
  when to avoid, 25
  who should, 25
  See also Exercises
Exercise diaries, 29, 30
Exercises
  for ankles, 35, 47, 92–93
  for arms, 37, 39, 48, 54–58, 98–101, 106–108, 113
  for back, 36, 37, 46, 47, 67–77, 109
  breathing, 34, 44, 122
  for calf muscles, 96
  cool-down, 98–101
  for elbows, 45, 55–58
  for eyes, 50
  for feet, 35, 92–96
  for fingers, 38, 39, 45, 61–64
  for hands, 38, 39, 60–64
  for hips, 36, 80–83, 110
  for jaw, 44
  for knees, 86–89, 111
  for legs, 36, 48, 96, 110–113
  morning wake-up, 34–41
  for neck, 37, 44, 50–52
  for posture, 46, 51, 52, 67, 69–70, 95
  for relaxation, 119–123
  for shoulders, 37, 39, 44, 45, 46, 54, 56–58, 106–108
  for stomach muscles, 72–73
  for thumbs, 60–64
  for toes, 35, 94
  warm-up, 43–48
  in water, 103–113
  for wrists, 60–61
Eyes
  exercises for, 50
  and rheumatoid arthritis, 4

Fainting, and aerobic exercise, 116
Fallen arches, 91–92
Feet
  arthritis in, 91–92
  exercises for, 35, 92–96
Fibromyalgia syndrome (FMS), 9–10
Fingers
  arthritis in, 59–60
  exercises for, 38, 39, 45, 61–64

Flexibility exercises, 24
Food Guide Pyramid, 16

Gold, as treatment for rheumatoid arthritis, 19
Gout, 15

Hands
    arthritis in, 59–60
    exercises for, 38, 39, 60–64
Headaches, one-sided, 49
Heart conditions, and aerobic exercise, 116
Heart rate, target, 116–117
Heat rubs, 20
Heels, tendonitis in, 9
High blood pressure, and aerobic exercise, 116
Hips
    arthritis in, 5, 79
    exercises for, 36, 80–83, 110
Hormone replacement therapy (HRT), 12
Hormones, and osteoporosis, 10
Hot water bottles, 20
Hypertension, and aerobic exercise, 116

Immune system, and rheumatoid arthritis, 3–4
Immunosuppressive drugs, 19
Insomnia, 33
Instep, 91–92

Jaw, exercises for, 44
Joint capsules, 2
Joints
    and ankylosing spondylitis, 7
    artificial, 20, 25, 79, 86
    and circulation, 43–44
    fusion of, 7
    inflamed, and exercise, 25
    and osteoarthritis, 5–6
    protection of, 20–21
    and rheumatoid arthritis, 4
    structures of, 1–2

Knees
    arthritis in, 5, 85–86
    bursitis in, 9
    exercises for, 86–89, 111

Legs
    exercises for, 36, 48, 110–113
    pain or numbness radiating down, 65–66
Lifting, 129–130
Ligaments, 2
    and ankylosing spondylitis, 7
Low-impact aerobics classes, 118
Lumbar spondylosis.

See Osteoarthritis
Lungs, and rheumatoid arthritis, 4
Lying down, on floor, 130

Massage, 20
Mattresses, 33
Medication, 18–19, 26
Menopause, and osteoporosis, 10
Mental attitude, 17
Morning wake-up exercises, 34–41
Motivation, 30–32
Muscles
    in joints, 2
    and rheumatoid arthritis, 4
    spasms of, in back, 66
    stiffness in, 9

Neck
    arthritis in, 4–5, 7–8, 49
    exercises for, 37, 44, 50–52
Nerves, and rheumatoid arthritis, 4

Occupational therapists, 19
Osteoarthritis, 4–7
    in hands, 59
    in lower back, 66
Osteoarthrosis. See Osteoarthritis
Osteophytes, 5
Osteoporosis, 10–13
    prevention tips for, 12–13
    risk factors for, 11

Pelvic rock, 69–70, 82–83
Penicillamine, 19
Pharmacists, 19
Physical therapists, 19
Pillows, 33
Poker back, 7
Posture, 50, 66, 126–128
    exercises for, 46, 51, 52, 67, 69–70, 95
Pulse rate, target, 116–117

QA. See Osteoarthritis
Quadriceps, 85, 86

Referred pain, 8, 49
Relaxation, 27, 119–123
    methods of, 120, 122
    and sleep, 122–123
Remittive agents, 19
Rheumatoid arthritis, 2–4, 25
    in hands, 59–60
    gold as treatment for, 19

Sacroiliac joint, and ankylosing spondylitis, 7
Sciatica, 65–66
Shoes, 24–25, 26, 86, 91
Shoulders
    arthritis in, 53

bursitis in, 9
exercises for, 37, 39, 44, 45, 46, 54, 56–58
tendonitis in, 9
Skin, and rheumatoid arthritis, 4
Sleep, 33, 35
    and relaxation, 122–123
Slipped discs, 65
Spine, arthritis in, 5, 7–8
    vs. sciatica, 8
Stair-climbing, 118
Standing up
    from floor, 130–131
    from sitting position, 128–129
Stomach muscles
    exercises for, 72–73
    and posture, 66
Strengthening exercises, 24
Stress, 17
Surgery, 20
Swimming, 25, 117
Synovial fluid, 2
Synovial membrane, 2

"Talk test," for exertion intensity, 116
Tendonitis, 8–9
Tendons, 2
    and rheumatoid arthritis, 4
    and tendonitis, 9
    and tenosynovitis, 9
Tennis elbow. See Bursitis
Tenosynovitis, 9
Thumbs
    arthritis in, 5
    exercises for, 61–64
Toes
    arthritis in, 5
    exercises for, 35
    tendonitis in, 9

Ulnar deviation, 60

Vertebrae, 49, 65

Walking, 117
Warmth, 20, 33, 104
Warm-up exercises, 26, 43–48, 117
Water exercises, 25, 103–113, 117
    guidelines for, 104
Water on the knee. See Bursitis
Weight, and arthritis, 15
Weight-bearing exercise, 12
Whiplash, 49–50
Wrists
    arthritis in, 59–60
    exercises for, 60–61
    tendonitis in, 9

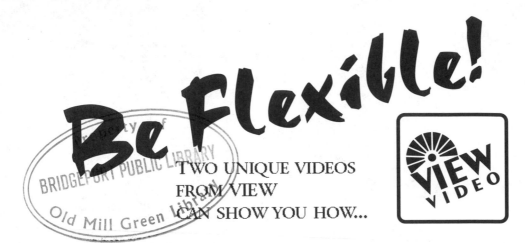
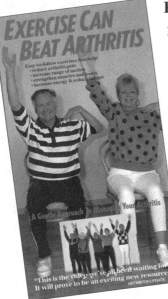
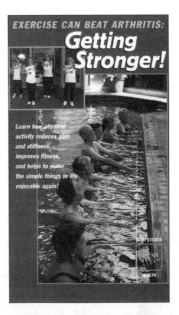